The Last Waltz
Love, Death & Betrayal

SEAN DAVISON

The Last Waltz: Love, Death & Betrayal

Author's Note & Copyright

The Last Waltz is a critical review of end-of-life options. It makes no recommendations about medical care. People reading this book must take full responsibility for their own health care. Accordingly, the author and publisher disclaim responsibility for decisions based on information contained herein.

All Rights Reserved

Copyright (c) 2015 Blue Danube Publishing

No part of this book may be reproduced or transmitted in any form or by any means, electronic or mechanical, including photocopying, recording, or by any information storage and retrieval system without permission in writing from the publisher.

ISBN # 978-0-9889691-7-9

Blue Danube Publishing

Printed in the United States of America

Designed by Elaine Feuer

First Printing

To order additional books, or to contact the author or publisher:

http://www.elainefeuer.com

elaine@elainefeuer.com

seandavison1@gmail.com

About The Author

In 2006, Sean Davison cared for his terminally ill mother, Dr. Pat Davison (a psychiatrist), during the final three months of her life. ***The Last Waltz*** is a true story about the extraordinary love between a mother and son, and how their informed decisions lead to unforeseen consequences: A sister betrays her brother; a son is charged with murder; Archbishop Desmond Tutu requests bail; igniting a public debate about voluntary euthanasia and the right to die in New Zealand, South Africa, and in countries across the Globe.

Sean has a doctorate in microbiology from the University of Otago in New Zealand, and is a Professor of Biotechnology at the University of the Western Cape in Cape Town, South Africa. He oversees the DNA Forensics Laboratory and has initiated a project to prove the innocence of people wrongfully convicted of crimes, by using DNA testing that was not used at the time of their conviction.

CONTACT SEAN:

seandavison1@gmail.com

The Last Waltz: Love, Death & Betrayal

Table of Contents

ABOUT THE AUTHOR	4
PROLOGUE	6
PART ONE: LOVE	9
PART TWO: DEATH	85
PART THREE: BETRAYAL	165
ARCHBISHOP DESMOND TUTU'S LETTER TO NEW ZEALAND HIGH COURT	238
PHOTOS	239

Prologue

I am feeling so much pain as I watch Mum slowly fading away. I wonder if this will have any lasting effect on me; I don't think so as I am emotionally strong, but it is very stressful. She just lies in bed all day waiting to die. It breaks my heart.

I don't want my Mum to suffer, so I must let her go. It is just so instinctive to try to hold on to someone you love as long as possible, but by doing that I am prolonging her suffering. Sometimes I feel she is holding on only because I am not letting her go. She is still giving me so much pleasure. Every time I am with her she gives me these beautiful, kind smiles. Today I asked her why she can smile so easily when she is suffering so much. She replied, "They are smiles for you."

It is becoming very difficult for Mum to walk to the toilet and I now have to escort her. She told me that she wouldn't need to go to the toilet during the night. However, as it turned out, at 4:30am I was woken by the sound of her dragging herself to the toilet on her own. This was no ballet performance; she was clinging desperately to each wall, trying to pull her frail body along. She had already made it past my bedroom door before I came and escorted her. She probably would have made it on her own, but it was a huge effort, and the potential for falling was high.

I am shocked at how frail Mum has become now. This is particularly noticeable when she tries to stand or walk. Her trips to the toilet symbolize her loss of independence more than anything else, and are

The Last Waltz: Love, Death & Betrayal

embarrassing for her. I have managed, however, to turn these trips into a playful ritual. When she needs to go I ask her if I can have the pleasure of a dance. I then lift her up so that she is standing only lightly on her own legs and announce which ballroom dance it will be. We then move together, in time to a fox trot, tango or waltz. When we get to the turn in the hallway, I lead her through a spin turn. She appreciates the fact that I take the dance timing seriously, not making a mockery of the circumstances. She taught me to waltz when I was a small boy; it is time to return the favor.

The Last Waltz: Love, Death & Betrayal

The Last Waltz: Love, Death & Betrayal

Part One

Love

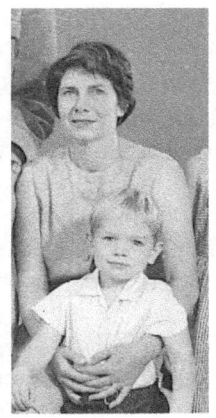

"Ae fond kiss"
Ae fond kiss, and then we sever
Ae farewell, alas, forever
Deep in heart-wrung tears I'll pledge thee
Who shall say that fortune grieves him
While the star of hope she leaves him
Farewell, thou first and fairest
Farewell, thou best and dearest.

Robert Burns

The Last Waltz: Love, Death & Betrayal

3 November 2004
Hotel Singapore

Mum could be dead now. If she is not, she could be dead by the time I finish writing this page. Or she could be dead before I arrive in New Zealand. This nightmare began yesterday with a telephone conversation. It was similar to the one described in the news when Rob Hall was stranded high on the top of Mount Everest in 1996. He spoke to his pregnant wife several times as he lay dying, waiting for his oxygen cylinder to run out. They had their last conversation, knowing that when they hung up that was the end, forever.

That was how I felt when I rang Mum after she had come out of the emergency operation on a tumor in her intestine. She told me she was certain she would not live until the morning, and therefore certain she would not live until I got there from South Africa. She said she would try very hard to hold on but it was out of her control because she felt she was at death's door.

I had no problem believing Mum's prognosis, for two reasons. Firstly, she is a very competent medical doctor who has dealt with dying people all her life, and, secondly, I've never known her to be sick or complain of any poor health. This last factor carried a huge weighting. When someone who is never sick tells you they are sick, you believe them. When this person is eighty-three and tells you they will be dead in the morning, you also believe them. When this person is your mother and you live ten thousand kilometers away you jump on the first available flight to get to them.

So I am now on my way to New Zealand. That dreadful conversation was yesterday. I told her I would be on a flight in the morning, and she told me she felt she wouldn't live to see me. She was even very apologetic about it, as she knew how much I wanted to be there. I told her how important she was in my life, how she had shaped me, how she was always the pillar of my life even when she was on the other side of the world, how nothing would ever be the same without her.

It was so difficult to put down that telephone receiver knowing it was probably the last time.

The Last Waltz: Love, Death & Betrayal

I phoned her as soon as I landed in Singapore tonight. She was still saying she didn't think she would be alive when I got there. We repeated much of what we said yesterday. This is such emotional torture. I accept that she will certainly die any day now. I just have one wish, and that is that she will live until I get there tomorrow.

TWO YEARS LATER

Wednesday 9 August 2006
Hotel Singapore

Again I am on my way back to New Zealand to visit Mum. Once again she is anticipating her imminent death. This time I am better prepared for it emotionally than that dreadful experience of nearly two years ago. I am ready to let her go this time; I just want to keep her company and make her last days happy. She seems very lonely when we chat on the phone, although she tries hard to hide it.

In each of our daily phone conversations we have mainly talked about whether she would have a visitor that day or discuss the callers from the previous day. These visits have seemed to be the only things keeping her going after her unexpected recovery two years ago. Most days she has no company and goes for a drive to the supermarket in the city just to have some human contact in the form of a supermarket checkout girl or a casual acquaintance. Recently, she lost the ability to drive as her right leg became weak and wobbly. Since then she has been forced to stay at home and this has changed her life dramatically.

Not only has she not been able to make those rather sad trips to the supermarket, but she hasn't been able to attend her art classes twice weekly. These classes have been the highlight of her week in the ten years since moving to Dunedin after Dad's death. She has also not been able to continue her weekly lunch appointment with Gwyneth or dinner at Richard's place. At least with Richard and two grandchildren, she has some family contact in Dunedin. Richard has been a dutiful son-in-law in the absence of any of her actual children. He has really performed beyond the call of duty in offering Mum help in every aspect of her life. I wonder if he has any unresolved issues to deal with following the suicide of his own mother when she was still middle-aged.

It seems so unfair that my mother should have four healthy, intelligent and caring kids and yet not have any of them around to take care of her at the end of her life. It seems that we are all so wrapped up in our own lives that we have left our own mother in our wakes, to die a lonely death. This is a cruel tragedy that I cannot let happen. I also feel in some ways that I am destined for the role. Mum has often said that she has always imagined she would spend her final years living with me. That prediction obviously hasn't happened, but at least that prophecy will now come true in her final hours.

I have jokingly told Mum that I am angry with her for summoning me to her deathbed at this time of the year. I have been telling her all year that the only month I could not come over was August because this is when I have a double lecturing load involving both Cape Town universities. She told me she had marked this on the calendar and would make every effort to stay healthy until after August. Sure enough, as August got closer and closer, Mum got more and more sick. First came the higher blood antigen counts from her colon cancer from two years ago, then the secondary cancer was found in her lungs, and then more recently in her liver and cerebellum.

So, following the rapid spread of her cancer, I began making plans to go back to New Zealand to be with her. Since Mum had no pain and was feeling no symptoms from these cancers, I decided I would go after I had finished teaching at the end of August. In the last two weeks, however, she has started feeling weaker and weaker by the day and has begun talking about not being able to survive until I arrive at the end of the month. When she became unable to drive, her feeling of total disempowerment and loneliness increased. Her demeanor in our daily phone calls is very pitiful, as she seems to be holding on from one day to the next in anticipation of my arrival, which seems so distant.

The Last Waltz: Love, Death & Betrayal

That's why I've felt I had no option but to book my tickets and get to New Zealand as soon as possible. I initially made a booking in the first week of August and kept delaying it day by day, so I could squeeze in as many lectures as possible before I left. Also, things are at such a critical stage in my research, I am nearly at the point of getting the South African Innocence Project up and running. It may be hard to sell this project to the public. I will have to explain it in simple terms because so many people are still unfamiliar and suspicious about DNA and what can be done with it. The project involves testing crime scene DNA samples that were not tested at the time a person was convicted, and this will only be in crimes where the convicted persons maintained their innocence. Many people in South Africa are surprised that I am initiating such a project to free prisoners when the crime rate is so alarming. They would much prefer to see more perpetrators who are walking the street convicted. I believe it is far more important to free an innocent man sitting in jail with a life sentence than to find the guilty man walking the streets. I am sure the South African community will also understand this after empathetically experiencing the suffering of the many anti-apartheid activists, such as Nelson Mandela, who cruelly and undeservedly spent decades behind bars.

Mum is also suffering cruelly, and the emotional pain of having Mum suffering on her own so far away, and the unintentional psychological pressure from her, became so great that I had no choice but to confirm my flight and leave for New Zealand.

Mum is quite certain that she has not got long to live. Of course I did hear this from her nearly two years ago, but this time she really has got all of the clinical evidence of advanced cancer and steadily declining health. It is impossible to believe anything other than an imminent death for her. Mum speculates that she only has a few weeks to live and refuses even to talk about her birthday in September, as she believes she won't be here for it and says that her life is becoming so miserable that she just wants it to end as soon as possible.

The Last Waltz: Love, Death & Betrayal

I am arriving in New Zealand tomorrow in the painful knowledge that I won't be leaving until I see Mum's body in a coffin.

Friday 11 August 2006

Mum was at Dunedin airport to greet me when I arrived today. I had already phoned her from Christchurch, where I had been stuck all day waiting for my domestic flight, so I knew something of her plan of how to get there. As she has not been driving, she arranged for my eldest niece to drop her off at the drop-and-go zone while my niece parked the car.

Mum was standing alone in the reception lounge. I was very surprised to see her there alone after what she had been telling me about her declining health, but she did look very frail. I took this as a good sign. Perhaps she was not as bad as I had expected. As is usual for her when her children are in airplanes, she was looking overly anxious. Once she caught my eye, her worries vanished into tears of joy.

I cried too. I have not done so before, but this time would be the last. The combination of these emotions and the exhaustion of a long flight were all too much for me to control.

But control myself I must.

We all get to bury two parents, if life takes its normal course.

I have watched several of my close friends suffering after the death of a beloved parent. I never really understood their pain, as I did not suffer greatly when Dad died. I am no different from my friends, and Mum's imminent death is no different from any other child's loss of a parent. I just have to keep reminding myself that it is inevitable. I must just bite the bullet and get through it and get on with life. It is only a matter of days or weeks now. Who knows?

From the airport we drove to Dunedin and dropped my niece off at Richard's place on Crosby Street, and then headed off towards Mum's home in Broad Bay. Finding myself in the driver's seat was in itself an adjustment. Throughout her life Mum has insisted on doing all of the driving, simply because she enjoys it.

The Last Waltz: Love, Death & Betrayal

In spite of all her driving experience, most people perceived Mum to be a dangerous and erratic driver. She did drive too fast and carried out many spontaneous and risky maneuvers, but whether this made her a bad driver or not is a debatable point. When my sister Mary was living in Dunedin, Mum used to help her out by fetching and dropping the kids off at their music lessons. But Mary eventually stopped this arrangement as she considered Mum's driving to be too dangerous for her children to be in the same car with. I am less critical as I see my own driving style in Mum's. I get the same complaints from passengers in my car, and since I feel in total control behind the wheel, I have come to the conclusion that Mum and I must both be good drivers.

On the way back home, Mum proudly told me that since she had stopped driving for life, it was now the time to make a final assessment of her driving ability and her driving record. She said that without having to "touch wood" she could say that she had had no serious accidents in sixty-five years of driving, and must therefore be considered a good driver, in spite of all the accusations that had been leveled against her by friends and family.

I couldn't argue that point.

On the way home we stopped at the New World Supermarket to stock up on food for me. Shopping has always been a highlight of my times with Mum, ever since I was a boy. I would always go to the supermarket with her, and without question get an ice cream. The joy of shopping with Mum is her incredible generosity, most noticeable with food, as her maternal instinct has always wanted to ensure we are very well fed – hardly noticeable, looking at our lean frames today. The more recent outings to stock up her house when we visit have become like those three-minute-trolley-grab prizes you win in competitions, but without the rush. Whatever we've wanted we've just tossed into the trolley. Mum never shows any concern about the price. She is interested only in seeing if we've bought something new to eat that she may enjoy too. We weren't spoilt children, in the sense of always getting our own way. It was just that Mum put so little value on material wealth. I think had she been in poorer circumstances, she would have found other ways of letting her generous spirit be expressed.

In addition to food, there's warmth. Sure enough, on the drive Mum checked with me that I have enough jerseys. As it turns out, this was exactly what had been going through my mind. It is quite a shock to move from the gentle climate of Cape Town to the depths of winter in Dunedin.

She really has been a wonderful mum to all of us. We don't give our parents much credit for their parenting until we are in the same position ourselves. Although I haven't had kids, I now marvel at how Mum managed. She held down a full-time job in various hospitals as the family moved around the world before finally settling in New Zealand, and at the same time she brought up four healthy children. She also had to deal with a rather difficult and demanding husband.

Her last full-time job, as a psychiatrist at Seaview Hospital, was very time-consuming. There were only three psychiatric doctors and one had to be on call at all times. Since Dad was the superintendent he was not expected to carry the same on-call work as his colleagues. Consequently, Mum had a heavy after-hours responsibility, and was often called out during the night.

But Mum loved working. Even after she retired from Seaview Hospital, she frequently did locums for the GPs in Hokitika, and I often heard from my former female classmates about how they always tried to see her. I imagine it was because they preferred going to a female doctor; throughout Mum's practicing days, medicine was very much a male-dominated field.

In spite of her workload she never really missed a beat in terms of parenting. She did occasionally have trouble getting to school prize giving and concerts. Twice as a boy I was near tears when Mum came dashing in towards the end of a school concert, long after I had given my performance on stage. I even remember catching her out when she tried to spare my disappointment by pretending she had arrived in time to see me.

Tonight Mum did not eat the food I cooked but instead made her own soup. We did this together, which is always enjoyable. Ever since I can remember, the kitchen has been the place for the most interesting interactions in our family. At least now we don't use the kitchen as a place to escape from Dad's stern gaze and authoritarian personality, and the very formally structured evening meals. It was always such a relief to get into the kitchen after dinner to dry the dishes, as we had such absorbing discussions in a happy environment night after night. I now wonder if Dad understood why the kitchen was such a happy place, and if he felt left out of the family bonding over dishes. I have still never had the honor of washing up after a meal. How long will Mum hold on to this monopoly?

Tonight I got the usual comment I get when I come home, about being too thin, and that I must eat more, especially meat. I told her that my weight has barely changed in twenty years and I had to blame my genes for the way I was built.

It seems that Mum is eating very little. She says she has soup every night because her appetite's so small, and soup has everything she needs. Tonight she had potato soup – really just boiled potatoes with lots of salt. Salt has always been a theme of her diet. It is sprinkled liberally on everything, and small bowls of it are to be found in several rooms of the house for her convenience. In spite of her overindulgence in salt, her blood pressure is amazingly normal. But it has always been a source of embarrassment to us when she orders extra jugs of water at a restaurant throughout the meal, to satisfy her salt-induced thirst.

Since I am so exhausted and jetlagged tonight I've decided not to discuss Mum's health, but just enjoy a relaxed evening with her, and write this journal. Tomorrow I'll go to the public pool, mainly to have a hot shower. Mum doesn't have a shower, and a bath in this freezing cold is unappealing.

As usual on these visits to Mum, we compare our use of Mogadon. She takes a tablet every night whereas I take half a tablet on rare occasions, when I desperately need to sleep. I will take a Mogadon for the next three or four nights to force my biological clock to get in synch with New Zealand time.

The Last Waltz: Love, Death & Betrayal

Saturday 12 August 2006

I had a solid eight hours' sleep last night courtesy of Mogadon. When I got up, Mum was already awake in bed, listening to the radio. She stays in bed until lunchtime most days, she says. She looked so comfortable and established there, I could hardly blame her. Her bed is littered with books, New Scientist magazines, crossword and sudoku puzzles, letters – it all seems a shambles, but she manages to find whatever she's looking for. I offered to make her coffee to save her getting up, and she was quick to accept. I was a little surprised by the concession, as I know she has the making of her morning coffee down to a fine art. Anyway, she gave me detailed instructions: in a saucepan, heat half a cup of milk and half a cup of water. I had to be careful heating the milk, she said, because you can't control the temperature on any of the oven-top plates. She made it very clear that I must never leave anything unattended for this reason (as if I couldn't work this out for myself). Once the milk is boiled, I should then pour it directly on to a teaspoonful of coffee in the cup, to scorch the coffee powder. Add a dash of cream and a heaped teaspoon of brown sugar, but do not stir. This is important, as she likes her first sips of coffee to be sugarless, followed by a hint of sugar as she drinks down, with a nice sweet swig at the bottom. Well, she seemed to be happy with my first effort, and I even had the honor of making her a second cup. I seized this opportunity to put in an extra large dash of cream because I was concerned about how little she ate last night.

I know exactly how she feels about her coffee being just right. I'm also a little obsessive about having the perfect cup. Coffee is such a wonderful, legal drug, and because I have it only once a day, it has to be perfect. I don't want to spoil the occasion by being disappointed. Unfortunately Mum drinks only instant and I use only ground beans, so we can't share the same high together. Mum has a percolator, but it's not much good because there's always sediment on the bottom. Also she doesn't have a microwave, so it is difficult to keep the coffee piping hot, which is another of my coffee obsessions. I really should go and buy a filter coffeemaker since this is such an important part of my day.

Post-coffee seemed like a good time to discuss Mum's health. She is never moody so there is no "bad time" to talk about anything. She is more than happy to do this. She says, quite simply, that her days are numbered, and that I need to be aware of this. She puts the loss of mobility of her right leg and arm down to the expanding tumor in her cerebellum, and although she isn't in any pain yet, she wants to die sooner, rather than later. Her life expectancy is very short, she says, and there's no point in grimly trying to hold on as long as possible. She plans to steadily reduce her eating so that, by becoming weaker, she'll have more control over when she dies. She spoke to me as if she thought I would be really shocked by what she was saying. She asked several times, "You do understand how I feel, don't you?" And, "You do agree with me, don't you?" I didn't feel shocked as her logic made sense.

Whenever I talked about anything in the future, she interrupted me, saying, "I don't want to talk about it." I asked her what we should do for her eighty-fifth birthday, and she again said, "I don't want to talk about it." I didn't push the point. I am not a medical doctor as she is, and I have to accept that she is probably right and believes she will die before her birthday. She is frail enough for me to believe it. I knew I was coming here to be with her when she dies, so I am confident that nothing during this time will shock me. To be with her at her death is the best way to lose a mother. But I have never been with a dying person before, so I don't know how quickly death comes. I guess Mum could die any day now. This is what she wants and I will accept that.

Sunday 13 August 2006

The coffee-cream dietary supplement is working well. I am increasing the doses and she doesn't seem to notice. I think this extra cream, plus the spoonful of sugar, together with the soup at night, and perhaps a snack during the day, should keep her strong for quite a bit longer. She is looking better today, and she also seems more mobile than when I first saw her.

It has crossed my mind that Mum might be hamming up her wobbly legs a little. She negotiates herself around the house, in slow motion, from one item of furniture to the next. She launches herself from a chair into the open spaces of the room, alights on the bookshelf, where she pauses, and then she's off again towards the arm of the sofa. She looks very graceful, almost like a ballerina. I am convinced that this is done as a performance to highlight her genuine lack of coordination.

Is it for my benefit? She really deserves a little sympathy over her present illness, particularly because Mary often tells her she is fine and has many more years to live. Perhaps Mum interprets this as Mary not acknowledging her illness. Mary has just passed her consultancy exams as a gerontologist – a specialist in the rigors of growing old. Medically speaking, she is in a good position to advise Mum on the state of her health and longevity, but as a daughter with a complex relationship with Mum, she gives advice that should be taken with caution. I think Mum feels she has to prove she is sick for anybody to believe it. In fact, it should be the other way round: since she has never been sick before, apart from her colon operation, we should really believe it now.

I met one of Mum's friends today, Doug Ogle. Doug's mother, Mary Ogle, was Mum's best friend in New Zealand until she died a few years ago. I remember how Mary Ogle lived near Mum when she was still working at Seaview Hospital and the two of them would drive to Greymouth once a week for shopping, and to Christchurch every few months for bigger shopping trips. Intellectually they were well matched and well read, and they talked non-stop when in each other's company, but their discussion was never superficial. In fact they discussed matters like politics, religion, art and philosophy effortlessly. Mary Ogle really was a fascinating lady. When she moved away from Hokitika to Timaru, I used to pop in for visits when I drove past her home. Time would always fly by, because she was so knowledgeable and interesting. Anyway, her seventy-year-old son, Doug, seems to have stepped into his mother's shoes and has formed a similar friendship with Mum. He is intelligent and well read and he and Mum can also chat away for hours.

I went swimming this afternoon, just after Doug arrived. When I returned, the two of them hadn't moved from their chairs and were still talking. I joined them for a while and then excused myself, saying I was jetlagged and needed to rest. In truth, I am not someone who relishes sitting around chatting for hours, but I'm happy Mum has a friend who enjoys this.

I have now changed my assessment of Mum's health. Although she is undoubtedly very frail, I can see a definite improvement since I've been here, and I don't think her death is as imminent as I originally thought. The dilemma I have is that I anticipated staying here for only a month or so, to give Mum company until her death. I now think it's possible that she could live into next year. It would be very difficult for me to stay away from work and my own home as long as that. It is not just the staying away that is an issue – what am I going to do here for so long? Certainly it is a pleasure being here with Mum, but can I really stay here indefinitely, when there is no telling at this stage how long she has? It's awful trying to speculate on when my mother will die, but I have my own responsibilities.

Monday 14 August 2006

I love Mum's hunger for news and knowledge. She has the radio on for most of the day for an endless stream of interviews, book reviews, and magazine programs. But whenever I come into the room and sit on her bed for a chat or coffee, she turns the volume down as a sign that she much prefers human company, except for the hourly news, when she's quick to turn up the volume to listen to the headlines. I did point out to her that the news is unlikely to change significantly from one hour to the next unless something very dramatic happens, which I guess is what she's hoping for. It's a habit she can't break, and it pleases me because it shows that she's still engaged with the real world: George Bush,

The Last Waltz: Love, Death & Betrayal

Iraq and global warming. When she loses interest, I'll get worried.

We drove into Dunedin today. Mum regularly reprimanded me for exceeding the speed limit, insisting there were hidden cameras everywhere. I kept assuring her that there weren't, because I know how to spot them. Our trip was for her appointment with her own doctor, Dr. MacDonald. It had been postponed so that I could be here for it, in my capacity as Mum's chauffeur, and so that a family representative could be kept up-to-date on the status of her health.

On the way Mum kept picking things off her clothes and throwing them away. I was concerned, since there was nothing there to pick at. I was getting a little irritated by this mindless action. When I asked her what she was doing, she replied that her hair was falling out and she was picking it off her clothing before she saw Dr. MacDonald. I assured her that her hair was *not* falling out, and suggested that she was imagining it. But she was insistent, and carried on.

Mum's friend Gwyneth was waiting at Dr. MacDonald's surgery, as had been arranged, so she could catch up with Mum at the clinic and meet me again. Like Mum, Gwyneth is a retired psychiatrist.

I escorted Mum into Dr. MacDonald's office so that she could lean on me while she walked. (I got the feeling that this was not entirely necessary.) Then I returned to the waiting room and chatted with Gwyneth while Mum talked to Dr. MacDonald alone. He wanted me to stay for the consultation, but Mum wanted to talk alone first. I was quite happy not to be there in the beginning, as Mum's a very modest private person and I'm sure she wouldn't feel comfortable discussing all the details of her failing body in front of me. After about fifteen minutes Dr. MacDonald came out and called me in to join them. He is a gentle, kindly man of about sixty. Apparently, he used to go drinking with Dad when he was a house surgeon at Greymouth Hospital thirty years ago. He treats Mum like a family friend.

The reason he wanted me there was to tell me the obvious: that Mum doesn't have long to live, although he couldn't say how long. It could be weeks – or months.

The Last Waltz: Love, Death & Betrayal

However, he felt it was time for me to tell my siblings to come and say their last goodbyes to Mum. He asked when Fergus, Mary and Jo had last been here, and when they would be coming again. I was polite and answered the way I was expected to. But Mum and I both know that the others aren't going to come rushing to say goodbye just yet.

My siblings are all aiming for a deathbed farewell. This scares Mum a little. She has already told me, since I've been back, that she knows she is supposed to have wise and meaningful final words, but she doesn't know what she's going to say. She has never liked being the center of attention.

This fear of attention and public speaking reminds me that she never formally retired as a psychiatrist from Seaview Hospital because she didn't want to have to give a farewell speech. And this was after about twenty years of service! She simply worked less and less, and quietly stopped. Her post was advertised and filled, and her work friends hardly noticed that she had officially retired. (At Dad's retirement party, he had to be carried home afterwards.)

But Mum did give a speech to Dr. MacDonald today. It was her standard one about wanting to die sooner rather than later. She said that her death was inevitable and so she didn't want it to be long and lingering. Dr. MacDonald was at pains to reassure her. There wasn't much else that he could say. After all, what can one say about a person who is not shying away from her death?

I then left Mum and Gwyneth in the car to chat while I went for a swim and a shower. The Dunedin pool is magnificent and a good place to escape to. With all of this talk and preparation for Mum's death, there's a lot which I need to escape from.

Tonight Mum didn't believe me when I told her that I couldn't find any pillowcases in the linen cupboards. She spent a long time hunting herself before agreeing with me. Tomorrow I will buy some.

The Last Waltz: Love, Death & Betrayal

Tuesday 15 August 2006

Today being Tuesday, Verna the cleaning lady came. And today being Tuesday, I had better remember to put out the rubbish tonight – one of Mum's preoccupations.

Verna's been coming every week for some time now. I know from our phone conversations that Verna's been one of her most important contacts and that Mum always looks forward to her visits. First, there's the anticipation of Verna's visit on Monday, and then an analysis of her visit on Tuesday. I couldn't understand the importance of this friendship as surely they have completely different interests. I was looking forward to meeting her to see what was so special about her.

Verna is about forty, kind and sincere, with a good mind, but not an intellectual. She's a part-time schoolteacher in the mornings, and cleans for people for extra cash in the afternoons. She didn't make much of an impression on me, but I didn't stay very long to get to know her.

I felt very uncomfortable having her come and clean when she could see that I was fit and able to do the job myself: she might be wondering whether I was too high and mighty or too damn lazy. I have this same discomfort with maids in South Africa. There, however, I can rationalize it as job creation. But New Zealand, by contrast, is such an egalitarian society that I feel ashamed at having a cleaning lady doing what I can do myself.

Mum tried to put my mind at ease by saying that she was only coming to help her change the sheets and do the washing, which she herself found difficult to do. But to escape the shame, I disappeared for a couple of hours up the hill behind Mum's place, to Larnach's Castle.

This hike goes through farms with sheep, cattle, and horses, along winding paths over green hills and then up through a forest to the castle. Along the way there are stunning views overlooking these green hills and forests, with the ocean on one side of the hill, and the wide, spacious harbor on the other. The walk was welcome peace. I went alone and saw no one. My mind is still very much focused on

The Last Waltz: Love, Death & Betrayal

how to make each day memorable and pleasurable for Mum. I don't want her simply existing, just waiting to die.

The other thing I'm dealing with is growing frustration at my predicament. I gratefully see Mum eating more and getting stronger and stronger each day, while knowing that the stronger she gets, the longer she will live, and the more certainty I have that I will need to return to Cape Town in the interim. If I go back for a few weeks, I will be able to get my life and job better organized to enable me to stay here for a much longer time. I'd also be able to apply for six months' leave from my work. I can't discuss this with Mum yet, as she's really enjoying my being here in the mistaken belief that I am staying until her death. I can see this is becoming a "Catch 22" situation.

After the hike I had lunch. I then met my old varsity friend, Ian, for our regular weigh-in that marks my annual trip to New Zealand. Once again my weight remains unchanged at sixty-eight kilograms, and his continues to creep up to eighty-five. The weigh-in began as a competition when we stood on the scales at a chemist's one afternoon twenty-five years ago and discovered that our weights were exactly the same. The origins of the competition were that we were both so skinny and both so very competitive that the goal of the competition was to put on weight. Initially it involved lots of trips to the gym for muscle building. The aim of the competition for Ian has now changed as he strives to shed the spare tier around his gut. I am still sticking to the original goal, however.

Tonight Mum and I prepared our own food in the kitchen together. Again Mum was having soup. Although it is fun in the kitchen with her, it can also be frustrating. We have both evolved rational, but distinct and different, ways of doing the same task.

Cooking's quite a complicated procedure – there's a lot to co-ordinate and streamline, and everyone has their own methods, peculiar to their personalities and their kitchens. I know I'm sometimes appalled when I see things done other than the way I would do them, either in someone else's kitchen or my own, and I have to check a reflex to offer advice or lend a helping hand.

The Last Waltz: Love, Death & Betrayal

I come to Mum's kitchen with my own way of doing things (which is based on sound logic and years of experience working in a science lab – which is similar to a kitchen), and this stimulates Mum to suggest better ways for me to do things, such as how to peel and prepare vegetables. I try to relieve the tension by initiating a healthy debate on why we do things the way we do them, elaborating on my logic for the way I myself do it. Mum enjoys this type of interaction and she gravitates to the kitchen whenever I am there to put in her two-cents' worth. We end up discussing anything, from which way one should or shouldn't slice the onions, to which way to point the prongs of cutlery in the drying rack.

Wednesday 16 August 2006

Each time I come back to Broad Bay I always ask myself how someone as travelled and worldly-wise as Mum could end up in such a remote region of the world.

The tiny village of Broad Bay is isolated on the Otago Peninsula at the lower end of the South Island. Compare this with Mum's exotic past. Her father was a Reuter's correspondent, and she spent much of her childhood and adolescence travelling Europe as her father was moved around. She attended schools in England, Switzerland, Czechoslovakia, and Austria. Then she did her honors degree in physics at London University, and her medical degree at Queen's University in Northern Ireland. Even after she met and married Dad, the travelling didn't stop. After Fergus and Mary were born Dad took the family to New Zealand where he served as a doctor in the navy for a few years. While they were there, Jo and I were born in Takapuna. The family then went back to England before finally immigrating to New Zealand permanently. All this travel was done by boat. I think Dad worked as a ship's doctor on some of the trips.

Tonight Mum and I went to Doug Ogle's for dinner. I prepared myself for a long evening as Doug has a tendency to talk a lot. But to his credit, at least he talks intelligently. I usually disappear when he visits, leaving Mum to provide him with her eager ears, but once she had accepted his invitation for dinner there was no escape.

Mum was reluctant to go but she had fallen into the trap that I often fall into, forgetting that New Zealanders tend to refer to the evening meal as "tea." When she accepted the invitation, that's what she thought it was, until Doug later phoned to confirm a time of 6.30pm.

I remember when I first arrived in South Africa and got an invitation for tea, I arrived late in the afternoon, bottle of wine in hand, expecting to be served my evening meal, much to everyone's embarrassment.

Anyway, Mum's curiosity got the better of her and she was keen to see inside Doug's house. But she gets very tired in the evenings, and would have preferred to sit at home and just relax with me.

I left Mum at one side of Doug's house while I tried to find out which door was the one meant as the entrance (it was far from clear). I came back to discover she had disappeared off around to the other side of the house. I wasn't happy with this, as she's unstable on her feet and I should have been there for her to lean on. Anyway, the evening was very pleasant and Mum had two bowls of parsnip soup (his wife had been told that soup is all Mum eats these days). It really was very good, and I don't even like parsnips. Mum also helped herself to a chicken drumstick, to everyone's surprise. Her appetite is definitely improving every day.

Let me analyze my dilemma. I suppose I am now feeling a little irritated that Mum got so sick in August when I was emphatic that this was the month that I couldn't come. To have to drop everything and rush out here when she is far from terminal, I do consider a little unfair. I know I shouldn't be angry with her; I must accept that she is very ill despite the big improvement we're seeing now. It just seems so bizarre that she was insisting that she didn't have long to go, and wasn't sure if she could hold on until the end of the month.

I guess I should also tell myself that if she was so desperate to get me out here, it does mean that she really needed the company and it's a good thing that I'm here. I must be positive and remind myself of all the years that I was

The Last Waltz: Love, Death & Betrayal

totally dependent on her, followed by a lifetime of love and emotional support; the very least I can do is be here now that she needs me.

Now that I am here, how do I organize my life in Cape Town so that I can stay longer? And what do I do while I'm here? Mum has a fairly comfortable day with regular visitors. She doesn't need me constantly, so I do have a lot of free time.

I'm in the process of getting Mum's phone connected to the Internet so that at least I can keep in touch with work colleagues in Cape Town. I could write a science paper. I will soon have exam scripts couriered to me for marking, and I can prepare my DVD lectures for next year. All of these are work tasks, however, and they are not going to cheer me up. The worst thing here is the cold weather. From the moment I get up until the time I go to bed, I am working hard at keeping warm. It's very different from Cape Town, and the weather is a huge part of my life. If the sun is shining it keeps me happy, no matter how bad the rest of my life may be. In Dunedin, the sun may be shining most days but the temperature rarely rises above forty-five degrees at this time of year, so it isn't easy to go outside and embrace it.

Alternatively, I must try to work out a plan to get my siblings involved. Mum should always have one of us here and be looking forward to the next one's visit, but I know that Mum is particularly comfortable in my company, so she may not like that idea. Yet, she also knows I have a job and a life in Cape Town.

I realize it will be a project in itself to get my siblings here. I have spoken to them all since I arrived. Fergus was quick to say, "Well done, Sean, I gather you're doing the heroic thing and staying until the end," the implication being that he wouldn't need to leave London.

And Jo said, "I'm glad you're here – it's impossible for me to get away from my new teaching job." That was a body blow. I had been thinking that as she lives in New Zealand, she's in a position to do the most to help Mum; whereas, in fact, she's offering the least.

Mary, when I asked if she could come out from Melbourne, said how much time she's already spent on Mum

The Last Waltz: Love, Death & Betrayal

– she was at Dunedin Hospital for a few weeks in June – and now she's so busy that it will be impossible for her to come out again until the very end. I'm not sure how she will know when the very end is going to be.

Anyway, here I am without any support, in a very cold town, in the middle of winter, with few friends and nothing much to do for the next few weeks or months, except watch my mother die. This may sound bleak. It is.

Thursday 17 August 2006

Today I got the Internet connection, which makes me feel a lot better. I was at loose ends and felt very isolated until today. Now I can connect with people and my work in Cape Town, and also have access to all the information that adds pleasure to my life.

And I can make international calls for next to nothing. I phoned Raine this morning, which was evening time in South Africa. She took this first free opportunity to give me a full account of the latest dramas in her new Chinese art business. Mum also spoke to her briefly. Because of her fascination and respect for Chinese culture, she seems delighted that I have a Chinese partner. Naturally she is hoping for some more grandchildren.

I again got hold of Raine on the phone late tonight, morning time in Cape Town. She said she couldn't hear all of my earlier calls as she was working with power tools on some construction. Carpentry is a passion of hers, and when she commits herself to something she gives it a hundred percent. It becomes quite an obsession until it's mastered, and then she moves on to the next interest. I first noticed this soon after I met her and she wanted to improve her English. (It seems to me that the Chinese can spend half a lifetime in an English-speaking country and still not speak it fluently; mind you, I wouldn't fancy my chances at Chinese.)

I am monitoring the weather in Dunedin versus Cape Town. The weekend forecast here looks scary – minus temperatures and nothing above forty-degrees degrees for the next five days. But today was glorious (relatively speaking), with blue sky and sunshine. I realize that it's important for me to have some life of my own, in addition to taking care of Mum. As she gets sicker I'm sure I'm going to get more and more absorbed with caring for her, and will need some mental relief from the task. However, it's still an option that she will go into a rest home or hospice despite her abhorrence of the idea of leaving home.

Today Mum discovered the two packets of Florentines that I brought with me from Cape Town. These have now been opened.

Mum says that having me here gives her an incentive to live. She said that before I came back she was desperate for visitors each day, but this was only to keep her busy until I came. I did wonder what my role was when I saw so many visitors coming and going, and all of the appointments lined up for the following week. It was hard to imagine how she could have been so lonely, nor could I understand why I was summoned so desperately.

The longer I stay, the longer I can keep Mum happy and the longer she is likely to live. I suspect she has a dilemma that's similar to mine. Does she look after her health by eating well because she is enjoying my company, and risk that by living longer I'll have to leave her for a time to return to South Africa? Or does she continue to want the quickest death possible, with my company till the end? This is not a good situation for her to be in, either. I suppose I must stick to my resolve to make every day happy for her. I can only speculate as to how things may deteriorate.

I am now seriously considering the possibility of returning to Cape Town for a month. It has become very clear to me that everyone (Mum's friends, my siblings, Dr. MacDonald) has the impression that I am staying here until the end. This has made Mum very happy. But this pledge was made when it looked as if she was about to die. What I now think I'll do is assess the decline in her health over the next couple of weeks. If it looks as if she is declining slowly, I'll go back to South Africa for a month or so, still constantly phoning her, and then return for her final weeks, or months. If she's declining quickly, I'll stay. It will be a hard decision to make, though. Being terminally ill, she is likely to get worse over the time I make my decision. Today I spoke to Jo and Fergus about their doing a combined six-week stint here, if I go back to South Africa. They intimated that they are able to do this. But Mum did say that she wants me.

I must keep swimming to preserve my sanity. And, the swimming pool is the warmest place in Dunedin. Today I swam while Mum had lunch with Gwyneth. When I was here in January, the two of them met up a couple of times. Mum was quite mobile then, and was telling me how Gwyneth spent her days going from one old lady to another, taking them out for their walks. It has become her mission in life to help these elderly people in their twilight years. Mum was analyzing her role in Gwyneth's life at the time, and concluded that she wasn't one of her ladies who needed the exercise and the company, but instead needed a friend to have a chat and lunch with. But now she's rapidly approaching the role we joked about, and Gwyneth could be taking Mum for weekly walks soon. I doubt whether Mum could bear that.

Mum bought some lamb chops at New World today. For a variation in her potato soup recipe she boiled the potatoes with one of these, which seemed like quite a complete meal. When she offered me some soup I accepted even though I have never been big on soups. Its simple flavors were very tasty. Later, when we were doing the dishes, she asked me how I could call myself a vegetarian when I had soup cooked with a chop!

I should have asked her why she bought only low-fat milk for her coffee when she poured in generous quantities of rich cream.

Friday 18 August 2006

I have stopped punishing myself by checking the Cape Town five-day forecast. There the sun shines tauntingly. I remember when I went to South Africa for the first time, in 1992, my main concern was that there would be too much sunshine for me to get anything done.

Over coffee with Mum this morning, I had to ask her not to talk to Truffle in the evenings after I've gone to bed. I was woken last night, as on other nights, by her lengthy discussions with her cat while she tidied up in the kitchen, the last thing before bed. She was very apologetic, saying she's been doing it deliberately just to let me know that Truffle had come in for the night and she didn't realize how quickly I fell asleep.

I've become that cat's manservant. I'm forever opening the door to let her in and out, feeding her biscuits by hand, and generally carrying her around while she dribbles all over.

To try to tempt Mum into eating more, I think I will make my favorite bread and butter pudding tonight. The savory dishes don't seem to be appealing to her taste buds anymore. I'll make quite a lot, because it keeps well for a week. When we have finished that, the next pudding's going to be a steamed one; suitably heavy for after swimming. Mum made steamed puddings a lot when we were kids. They were called Sussex Puddles, and were made out of suet. I reminded her of this, and we both agreed that the idea of suet in a pudding nowadays is a bit revolting. She said that, in her childhood, her mother would go to the butcher to ask for suet, which was the solid fat cut from the animal. She would then take it home, wrapped in paper, and chop it up to make the Sussex Puddle pudding with a lemon cooked in the middle.

Mum came up with a new idea this morning. She said that since she doesn't stir the sugar once it's added to the cup, she'd like colored sugar so that she would be able to see the sugar intensity gradient in her coffee, from the bottom to the top. I wonder why nobody has come up with this idea before.

Tonight I moved my laptop to the kitchen, to be more sociable. It is more comforting for Mum to be able to see me even if I'm not directly interacting with her. Mum couldn't resist coming to the kitchen and finding something to do while I was there. Of course I didn't mind, although I couldn't concentrate very hard. She asked me what I was doing. I told her I was writing my diary. She asked if I was concerned someone might find it and read it. I said that was not a problem since it is an electronic diary and I keep it well hidden in obscure folders and files. She asked if I brought these folders and files all the way from South Africa. When I told her that they were in the computer she looked a bit perplexed, and then resigned herself to the fact that the electronic age had left her way behind in its wake. I imagine there are many elderly people out there who can perceive folders and files only in terms of cabinets.

Mum really has no excuse for not keeping up with the computer age. She is a mathematical genius, always with a supply of those problem-solving books, with titles such as *Games for the Super-Intelligent*. Never did a problem beat her. Her favorite pastime is doing crossword puzzles, and her standard Christmas or birthday present from us was a more challenging crossword puzzle book. She used to send in *The Press* competition crosswords, but after she won a few she submitted them under her children's names. I remember giving her IQ tests when I was at high school. I would explain that she had thirty minutes and had to work through the questions as quickly as possible. Mum would do the test just to humor me, but during the test she would get up and turn over her Bach symphony record, or even trim a dying leaf on one of her pot plants. No matter how many distractions there were she would always score a Mensa qualifying IQ of around one hundred and sixty.

She inherited her mathematical genius from her mother, who received a mathematics degree with honors at the Cambridge University. She also received several "first in class" distinctions. This was at a time when mathematics was a male-dominated field, and quite probably her mother was the only woman in the class. Of course, once she finished University she adopted the profession of wife, mother and housekeeper, as was expected in those times.

Unfortunately these math genes were not passed on to us kids. Although we are good at science and medicine, none of us inherited her natural flair for math. Mum, who practiced as Dr. Pat Ferguson, has always said that I took after her father, Fergus Ferguson, in so many aspects of my personality and character. Although her father showed no mathematical tendencies, he was still a high achiever, receiving a CBE from the King of England for his services to journalism as a Reuter's correspondent in Palestine, and awards for his coverage of the post-Second World War Nuremburg Trials.

Mum is still with me in the kitchen and is making a fruitcake. She asked if I would cream the butter and sugar for her, as her arms and wrists were not up to it. I told her that I had once seen an electric mixer in one of her cupboards and it would be very easy to do it with that. She said Mary had given it to her and she had since given it away unused, as she preferred baking the old-fashioned way. I didn't want to make an issue of it since it crossed my mind that this could be the last cake she makes, so I obliged. My wrists are still aching.

It was quite entertaining to watch Mum put the cake together. She had a good dozen handwritten recipes for the same cake, with different variations of the ingredients or cooking time and temperatures. The top copy was her working recipe, one that had obviously been fine-tuned to perfection. The way she put the cake together, however, seemed very haphazard. She just tossed in cups and spoons of ingredients without using exact measures. When the cake was cooked it was indeed delicious.

Saturday 19 August 2006

I didn't sleep well last night, but I'm determined not to get into the sleeping pill habit. If I start taking them regularly, there's the chance I won't be able to give them up, because generally I haven't been sleeping well.

I suppose this contributed to my intense irritation with Mum about her idiosyncrasies with the telephone. She insists on having a phone with a very long cable, rather than a portable phone like the rest of the world. This damn phone cable is a constant source of frustration because she keeps the phone on or near her bed, and has to negotiate the cord whenever she moves around the room. With her unstable legs, it's only a matter of time before she trips over it and takes a fall. The cable's connection to the wall isn't secure, either, so when the cable comes loose the phone doesn't work. Although this happens only occasionally, Mum indulges in thinking that it happens all the time. Basically, if anyone tells her they couldn't get hold of her, she puts it down to the dodgy cable. I've heard her explaining this to numerous friends on the phone. My own investigation

The Last Waltz: Love, Death & Betrayal

suggests that this is not the problem. Instead, Mum doesn't hear the phone ringing when she's in the bathroom.

This morning I tripped over the cable. I was okay, but it totally destroyed the connection inside the phone. As soon as I told Mum she gave me instructions to get a new one straightaway. I could understand her concern because before I arrived she'd been completely dependent on it. It's her connection to the outside world – for company, or if anything goes wrong.

Because she's not concerned about economy any more, she was intent that I drive into Dunedin and buy a new phone and connect it before I headed off for the day. My preference was to go into Dunedin, do all my own errands as planned, and return with the new phone later in the day. But for Mum, every hour without a phone is very stressful, and I realized I had better go and get a new one without further ado.

Although I know she was justified in her insistence, my irritation showed as I left. On the drive in I did actually kick myself to remind myself I must never show any reluctance again in response to requests she makes. Her days are numbered and she should have whatever she wants, no matter how inconvenient. I had no right to tell her that she didn't really need a phone for the day.

Once I'd got back an hour and a half later, and had the phone connected, I could see she was much more relaxed, and we were both making an extra effort to be especially friendly. She either felt guilty for asking me to make a special trip into Dunedin, or just felt bad at seeing me irritated with her. The lesson was probably a good one for both of us.

Apart from the phone episode this morning, Mum's been fine today. Saturday is her favorite radio day when Kim Hill, the presenter, has a half-day show on national radio. Mum's tossing back all the hot drinks I bring to her bedside: sweet creamy coffee, Marmite soup (she has gone through a whole jar of Marmite since I've been here) and potato soup. She even tried the cream liqueur I got for the bread and butter pudding last night.

I see the top temperature in Dunedin next week is going to be thirty-six degrees. This is one of the coldest winters

The Last Waltz: Love, Death & Betrayal

recorded in New Zealand. Today, there's a parade of topless women on motorbikes in Auckland. What are they thinking?

It will be nice to get out of the house and watch rugby with Ian this afternoon. I have seen him only once since I have been back as he's an hour's drive away.

Later the same day

It was a tri-nations game. All Blacks versus Ozzie, and the All Blacks crunched them! After that we went back to Ian's place to watch basketball. He took the opportunity to proudly show me the racing bicycle he bought last year. He said he had been in regular training to keep his weight under control. I couldn't resist pointing out the covering of cobwebs, but he was quick to assure me that he had been recovering from a bit of an injury, recently.

I phoned Mum to check that she was okay and to let her know that I'd be late. This was about 7pm. She said there was no hurry, as Richard and some of his friends had dropped by at five, after playing golf, and had made themselves comfortable on the couch.

Although I still hadn't seen Richard since I arrived, I wasn't in the mood for polite conversation tonight and decided to wait as long as I could before returning home, to give him time to leave. I phoned Mum again at ten, and Richard was still there. But because I was so tired, I thought I'd better go home.

When I got back at eleven, Richard and company were still there. Apparently, they'd been sitting on the couch for six hours, drinking wine, eating what they could find, and chatting to Mum. She seemed to be absorbed in their discussions, and was very happy. She is an attentive listener and one of Richard's friends seemed to be a skillful conversationalist. I was amazed that Richard's three friends could sit there and chat for seven hours (it was midnight by the time they left) with someone they hadn't met before.

Even though I had been reluctant to catch up with Richard, tonight, it was actually really good to see him again. He is such a dependable and stable influence in the family. Rather uncharacteristically, he asked me to teach him the basic steps for a tango, because he has been invited to a ball next week by one of Dunedin's leading socialites, Elizabeth Ellis. I put a daffodil between my teeth and led him through the basic steps, much to the delight of our tipsy audience.

I am very pleased that Richard has stayed such a big part of our family even after his divorce from Mary. Divorces are never pleasant and he could have easily disappeared off the radar, and we'd all have been the poorer for it.

Sunday 20 August 2006

Mum really is looking better by the day. She is smiling and happy and eating more. I found signs of nibbling when I got up this morning and came across half a chocolate brownie muffin in the kitchen. I certainly don't eat brownies in halves. Each morning she says she is feeling really good. Surely feeling good is reason enough to live? And she certainly hasn't lost the instinct to look after the stove. Often she imagines that I'm leaving saucepans on the top element unattended. Each time I have to assure her that I have things under control, and that I'll never let the coffee milk boil over.

Most of her friends have commented to me on how much she's improved since I've been here. They say that before I came she kept talking about when I was coming, and how much she was looking forward to it. Although Mum had chosen to decline all treatment for her cancer, she decided to have this radiotherapy to prevent her brain from turning "into cheese." Mum believed that to lose her mental faculties would be the worst possible way to go.

She's still paranoid about her hair falling out as a consequence of the treatment. But in spite of her insistence that it is, I can't see any evidence. She has always had strong thick hair. At the moment, though, she wears a home-knitted beanie, which means I don't get to see her head so often. She looks quite elegant and arty in these knitted hats. I realize that a woman's plumage is really her crowning glory, and to lose it would be devastating. A man is lucky. If he has a full head of hair he looks young and virile, if he has no hair he looks as if he has excess testosterone, and if he has half a head of hair he can shave the other half off. He is a loser only if he does a "sweep" combing a tuft from one side over to the other.

The district nurse came today and spoke to Mum in private. Nonetheless I thought it important to have an ear to the door, as I really need to know what Mum's thinking but not telling me. Sadly, she was saying to the nurse that she wants to die quickly – because of all the inconvenience she is causing her children. That's a terrible reason. I am now making it very clear to her that I am happy to be here.

The nurse told me that Mum has a strong heart in spite of the cancer spreading and speculated that she could very well have many months to live. I don't think she should be living alone in her frail state, gliding along the walls as she does. It's scary to contemplate. Although she has visitors nearly every day, they fill only a small part of the time. If I do go back to South Africa for a while I will do so only when another family member is here.

Later the same day

It's nearly midnight, and Jonah has just left. Apparently she's a regular Sunday night visitor. She comes and plunks herself on the floor in front of Mum's fire, puffs away on a joint and drinks a glass of wine.

Jonah is an unusual character. She's unemployed but has a collection of ex-lovers, who seem to take good care of her. She is now looking after a friend's house at the end of the Aramoana Tidal Spit.

She makes a big deal of being able to visit only when the tide is low, as she claims her house is cut off from the mainland when it's high. Mum thinks this is unlikely, and that Jonah uses it as a colorful excuse for when she fails to pitch up, or is later than she planned. Who can argue unless they've kept an eye on the tides? She is very good company because she is a little wacky and is a constant source of bizarre information.

The Last Waltz: Love, Death & Betrayal

Monday 21 August 2006

I no longer feel so despondent and I have stopped cursing my predicament. Mum's health has improved quite dramatically, and I have established a comfortable routine. I am adapting to life here.

Each day begins serenely with Mum's cup of coffee, accompanied by the daily reminder not to let the milk boil over, and my assurance that it won't ever happen. I do my emailing for most of the morning, then lunch and coffee with Mum (although the little she eats hardly constitutes a lunch), then into town and swim, or hike up to Larnach's Castle. In the evenings we settle in front of the TV. Although Mum has never been big on TV, she says it should be a social occasion. She enjoys it only if there is company. Because we get very little British TV in South Africa, I check the *TV Times* here each day and select the interesting British programs for us to watch that night. We both enjoy the murder mysteries – "Midsummer Murders", "Murder in Suburbia", "Rosemary and Thyme", along with a steady supply of British documentaries. We analyze the story together during the commercial breaks. Since Mum doesn't watch much TV, I often have to explain what is going on.

When I hiked up the hill behind Mum's place this afternoon, it felt really good. I realized that I'm now just as happy here as in South Africa. It's relatively stress free. In fact, with all the hiking and meditative swims, I feel as if I'm on a Buddhist retreat.

I do, of course, worry about Raine living on her own in Cape Town, but she assures me that she feels safe, and although she is missing me she understands my need to stay. She did say that Caesar and Cleo are probably less forgiving of my deserting them since she doesn't give them the long mountain walks they are accustomed to.

I now ask myself if there is any need to go back to South Africa. It will cost a lot and it's also a long trip for what would be a short time only. Each day with Mum is enjoyable. She talks freely about death and these talks are enlightening, rather than depressing. Her main concern is that she's going to die slowly. She had thought she was dying quickly, and she's disappointed to discover that she's not.

Richard has tried several times to coordinate with my nieces to come here together for dinner. He is going to try again tonight. It seems to be a project on its own to coordinate these girls. They seem a little preoccupied with the next distraction. I think Richard will cook. If not, I'll just knock up another pizza.

Mum is still fastidiously picking imaginary hair from her clothing. This irritates me, as there's no hair on her clothing and it's not falling out.

I did it again. I made the mistake of looking up the five-day forecast for Cape Town and discovered that every day is seventy degrees or more. By contrast, every day in Dunedin is going to be below forty degrees. I am waiting for the forecast snow to come. It's miserable today.

Mum had more visitors this afternoon. I'm off for a swim and of course a long hot shower. Then to chop some firewood afterwards; it's so very cold.

Tuesday 22 August 2006

Last night Richard managed to round up only one of my nieces to come for dinner. It is hardly surprising. He brought steak, his trademark dish, and it was great to see Mum tucking into it. I said in the future that, to make things easier, I'll cook when he comes here and he can cook when we go to his place. He liked that idea.

Mum and I spent a pleasant evening in front of the TV, watching British dramas. Because it was Tuesday night, we had our regular debate about putting out the rubbish. Mum likes it to go out on Tuesday night for its collection about nine on Wednesday, simply because we might forget about it in the morning. My own preference is to take it out on Wednesday morning, mainly because it is warmer then and also because we can include extra rubbish. She let me have my way tonight because it was so cold. There are other inflexible habits of hers with the rubbish that concern recycling, but that's another long story in itself. Mum is a passionate environmentalist.

The Last Waltz: Love, Death & Betrayal

Wednesday 23 August 2006

While I was making Mum's coffee this morning, I suddenly remembered to take out the rubbish. As I sifted through it and scrambled around outside, I lost track of making the coffee and the milk boiled over. I didn't notice this until I saw the smoke-filled kitchen and Mum called out in synch, "Have you left the milk on the hot plate?"
"All under control Mum"....grrr...

Mum was right. Her hair *is* falling out. I feel a little guilty for not believing her when she kept picking the strands off her clothes. I really thought she was imagining it, but it was hard to know with her wearing her woolen beanie. Last night I watched her burn handfuls of hair in the fire. She seems to be taking it in her stride, but for me it's quite a shock. I wonder if it will all fall out.

Thursday 24 August 2006

Thursdays have become Gwyneth days. I quite like these landmarks in the week. It gives Mum something to look forward to most days. As usual, we drove into town with Mum regularly reminding me not to speed because of the hidden cameras everywhere. This time I could categorically tell her that she was being paranoid. I had read in the local newspaper that Dunedin has only three fixed speed cameras, and there surely aren't any on the road we use. If there were, we'd see them. This didn't stop Mum.

Once again I left her with Gwyneth at the Nova café in the Octagon and went for a swim. Afterwards, I had a quick bowl of soup with them before Mum and I continued on our expedition. We went for a drive up North East Valley and had a look at the hospice from the outside. When I was in here in January I went on a tour of the place with Mum and Jo. We had laughed afterwards when we were outside, because it seemed so obviously not the place for Mum – sterile and clinical, with a pious guide who spoke in hushed whispers. There was no way we could dream of putting Mum in there. Funny and sad how things have changed, now that it's a possibility.

The Last Waltz: Love, Death & Betrayal

Since then Mum's been back to visit the place with Mary, and now has a more favorable impression. She's considering a rest home or hospice if I have to go back to Cape Town. I have acknowledged that this is a possibility, but I've also told her that I'd arrange for Mary, Jo or Fergus to fill in the gap while I'm away. She's clearly unhappy at the prospect of a rest home.

We then stopped off to do the shopping at New World. I was surprised that she didn't want to come in, but preferred to wait in the car. She's always loved shopping for groceries, so I took this as a sign that she was very tired. It felt strange doing the shopping without her.

On the way home I took her on a drive around the peninsula. At her request we went past a rest home where I parked outside for a moment. She looked so very sad as we sat in the car, looking at this unwelcoming building. She mumbled that this area seemed nicer than North East Valley. I could feel her agony even though she would never express it. She felt that the people she cared about so much no longer wanted her around. They would put her in a home full of people she had nothing in common with except they shared a similar age.

I returned to have a look inside that old people's home after I took Mum back. The nurse at reception was very happy to show me around, gave me a brief tour, and then left me to look around on my own. I sat and chatted to an elderly lady who was knitting a jersey. Was it for one of her grandchildren? "No," she said. "No one cares about me since I was dumped here. Do you want a jersey?" I politely declined.

When I spoke to the nurse on the way out she said, "It's basically a dumping ground. It breaks your heart. People phone and say, 'Do you have accommodation? How much? I'll pay anything if you'll take them. I can't cope anymore!' They drop the parent off and promise to visit, and a few do, but you don't see most of them for weeks . . . or ever."

Apparently the old people are in shock, left among strangers, embarrassed to need bathing and nappies – stripped of their dignity in the last days of life. Some die within weeks. I was told that one old woman carried a brick around with her. At night she'd hide it in the garden and say goodnight to it. I think if I were forced to live in this place I would also be carrying a brick from my old home around with me.

The elderly are the lifeblood of any society, yet we conveniently forget them. If only we realized while we are young what could happen to us in old age, at least it would help us make plans. Look at the situation Mum has found herself in. She just assumed everything would work out all right for her. Perhaps it will.

Some may say that we should have put Mum in a place like this. They'd say that few elderly parents like the decisions that are really best for them. But no, Mum made the right decision to stay at home, and we were right to respect her wishes.

I'm sure most people take the last surviving parent into their own home in their final years. We should have done that in our family. I regularly asked Mum to come and stay with me in Cape Town. She had always said she thought she would end up living with me in old age, but the reality of living in a very hot climate ruled me out. I don't think Jo was an option since they were not particularly close. Fergus lived in England and Mum probably didn't contemplate moving there. The obvious answer was Mary in Dunedin. About six years after encouraging Mum to move to here after she was widowed, Mary had left to live in Melbourne. Mum felt abandoned by her, but I don't blame Mary. It is a bit unfair for any child to be forced into adopting their parents in their old age when they have their own families and careers to consider. On many occasions over the past two years Mum has mentioned moving to Mary in Melbourne to end her days, and possibly going into a hospice there. She knew she wanted to be near family when she finally died.

One of the reasons Mary left New Zealand was because of her association with a Dr. Bowen, a now jailed South African doctor who poisoned his wife. Mary was having a relationship with him in Dunedin and was taken into custody with him at the time of his arrest. In the subsequent and high profile court case it was revealed that Mary's signature was on the prescriptions to get the poison that killed his wife. It was later learnt that he had been forging Mary's signature. Everyone knew Mary's association with Dr. Bowen, even though her name was suppressed. I gathered from Mum that this doctor was very charming and that Mary was head-over-heals in love with him, and she knew nothing about the murder at the time. I didn't learn about this until long after the event.

We drove along the top of the peninsula with all its magnificent views, and stopped at a sheep farm where they sell homespun wool and knitted jerseys. Mum buys a jersey for me every time I come home, as a present and a tradition. I chose a jersey with large brown checks in dark and light, although Mum's first choice was a plain light grey one.

We got home by five, so that I could prepare dinner for Richard and the nieces he was going to round up. I couldn't reach him by phone and left a message on voicemail, asking him to confirm when he'd be here. I already had the pizzas in the oven when he phoned at six-thirty to say they weren't coming for dinner after all, and that he'd been trying to get hold of us. He suggested that the phone wasn't working, availing himself of Mum's dubious telephone excuse, not realizing we had a new one. The real reason is that he hadn't tried hard enough.

Mum has an affectionate nickname for Richard behind his back. It's "Either-Or." Because he seems to be incapable of making a fixed plan, it's always, "either this, or that," making it difficult for everyone around him to coordinate anything. After tonight, I've vowed never to prepare dinner for Richard until he's actually at the house.

Mum's in agreement with this new strategy. I rather appreciate her maternal protection and must enjoy it while it lasts.

Friday 25 August 2006

Mum enjoyed the bread-and-butter pudding the other night, although I thought it was a bit stodgy. I'll make another one tomorrow, but this time I'll leave the bread to soak in the egg, milk and Amarillo.

The Last Waltz: Love, Death & Betrayal

Tonight I gave Mum a real treat by taking her on an Internet tour, using the Google Earth site. She was quite blown away by the technology. She sat glued to my computer as I took her on a satellite tour of all her children's neighborhoods, plus her own. At one point in the evening Mary phoned, and I told her that we were looking for her house in Melbourne. She gave me instructions over the phone as I navigated around the streets in her area. Mum's eyes were popping out as we did this. Once I'd found her house, I told Mary to stick her arm out her window, so we could be sure it was hers. I then said I could see it. Mum couldn't see Mary's arm, but she believed it.

Technology has moved light years since her days as a radar operator during the Second World War. At that time she was right at the cutting edge of science, and physics in particular. Mum used her physics training during the war to operate radar tracking of the German missiles bombarding London, and her team of physicists were responsible for designing the strategy for blocking German radar by the aerial dropping of tin foil over Berlin in the latter stages of the war.

Mum sat beside me for the better part of two hours as I continued to "surf" the Internet. I explained what I was doing and all the information I could access at the push of a button.

At one point I introduced her to Wikipedia and explained that this online encyclopedia is now one of the world's top ten websites, unique in that anyone who logged onto it could create, write, and edit entries on any subject that struck them as worthy. It had changed the way much of the world gets its information.

When Mum asked if I used it, I explained that it was difficult to avoid since it automatically presented itself when one does any word search on Google.

She said, "But what's wrong with using the *Encyclopedia Britannica*?"

I told her that it was just a little out of date, and is fixed in time, whereas Wikipedia is constantly being updated. Such an argument didn't hold much sway with Mum, who still uses her 1911 edition!

The Last Waltz: Love, Death & Betrayal

She was adamant, "That is its strength. Time gives the writers a chance to consider their ideas and acquire a little perspective." She continued, "It is beyond my comprehension. There seems to be no authority or authenticity in an encyclopedia that is written by the people who are reading it."

I left it at that.

Against my better judgment, I decided to introduce her to Facebook. I showed her a page and explained how this was becoming one of the most popular means of communication for the young. She looked aghast when I told her that studies show it is now becoming common for parents and children to communicate by this method.

We continued our journey as I took her to YouTube and a few other modern sites. She occasionally asked questions, which revealed how new this was to her. I could see that she was struggling to decide whether to embrace modern technology or just let it pass her by. Life was so easy without it. It must be very unnerving to be old and to gradually see the world, as you know it, recede out of existence. It's hardly surprising she doesn't want to leave the sanctuary of her own home.

Technology has not just increased life expectancy but has stretched the generation span. Old people are now being increasingly sidelined. It is almost as if a new class of people have emerged who are too old to keep in touch with change. This is accentuated by the speed at which changes are happening. Show me any grandmother who really understands her grandchildren and their rapid electronic communications culture.

When I retired to my room for the night I was still fresh enough to tackle the exam marking which arrived by courier today.

Saturday 26 August 2006

Today I got Mum to sign some of her paintings that I brought back from Cape Town, in addition to a new bundle I acquired today. I told her that I wanted them initialed because, as with many artists, her extraordinary talent may be discovered only after her death. She scoffed at this suggestion. I was quite surprised that she was willing to do this, however, when she is so modest about her works and never voluntarily shows them to anyone, nor has any on display in the house.

After she initialed them all I realized the initials in the bottom corner were too low down and would be lost once I framed them, so I asked her to initial them all again higher up. Again she was more than happy to humor me. This process took a good hour as I had quite a pile of mostly sketches. It was also very interesting listening to her commenting on the subject matter, or the circumstances behind many of the paintings. The self-portraits drew some very damning comments.

When Mum and Dad moved to their retirement house in Kaniere, Mum had only one request, for a room to be built on to the house with no connecting door. At the time I assumed this was the essence of being an artist, having a space to let your mind be free, to think any thoughts, and let your brush be the expressive force. Mum spent many hours in this room and constantly pushed her artistic expression to the limit. It is so evident with artists that the beauty of their creative works lies in their striving. Now I spend more time on reflection, I know exactly why she was so emphatic about having a separate granny cabin. It was to have a place to escape from Dad's tyrannical rule.

Sunday 27 August 2006

Saturdays and Sundays are the days Mum's fellow art class students visit. There is a certain irony in her attending classes when she has been painting for at least forty years. I even recall she did School Certificate and University Entrance exams at Westland High School after I left there. She was just determined to get as much practice as she could. The school students were quite bemused having a seventy-two-year-old studying with them.

So it's been a weekend of visitors. Mum has some wonderful friends who really seem to love being with her. The amazing thing is that these are all people she's met since

The Last Waltz: Love, Death & Betrayal

she arrived in Dunedin. They've known her only as an elderly lady.

The first of the weekend visitors is always Norton. He's a retired mathematician his eighties, whom Mum met at art classes. He's exceptionally bright and knowledgeable and comes to visit Mum each Saturday with a muesli bar he buys for her at the Dunedin produce market. It's become a ritual.

This weekend he asked for a photo of Mum and me, from which to paint us. I obliged with one I'd taken last week; it's of the two of us sitting together on her couch. I apologized for the fact that the old dying mother had a more beautiful smile than the young son with a full and exciting life ahead of him. Norton replied, "It's because the mother knows she is in the company of a son who loves and cherishes her."

Peter Hinds pops in periodically on Sundays. He's a retired doctor, also in his eighties and from art class. He brings his latest "works in progress" for Mum to give advice and comment on. Today he brought his painting of a witch on a broomstick crashing into a telegraph pole. Peter, having been a doctor, is practiced at being concerned and wise. Each time he visits, he makes a point of talking to me alone in the garden. He checks that I'm holding up okay, and invites me to come and see him in town if I ever need to talk about the difficulties I'm having looking after Mum, but I feel I am coping fine.

John Francis also came today. His modus operandi is to phone a few days before he comes, to say he'll visit as soon as he gets some money for petrol. I'm not sure if he's hinting that I should buy it for him. John is a very widely known and eccentric artist in Dunedin. In spite of the popularity of his art, I'm ambivalent. Yet I must respect the fact that Mum thinks the world of it. Sometimes he stops along the road on the way and does a sketch which he then presents to Mum on arrival. Today's sketch looked like little more than scribble on a page. Initially I thought he was pulling my leg, but once he started explaining the deep profound meanings of this work I realized I had to keep a straight face.

And of course Jonah came tonight. Which means it must have been low tide. Jonah's only association with the art group is that she occasionally strips for them. She brought a

The Last Waltz: Love, Death & Betrayal

homemade spinach quiche and presented it to us with a string of apologies: the pastry had been sitting in her fridge for weeks, the cheese had gone off but should be okay, the spinach was growing outside her garage and was almost dead, but it should be all right, too. She called it a "happy quiche." It certainly tasted unusual. Mum and I discreetly discarded our portions into the compost bucket when she wasn't looking. Jonah seemed to enjoy it, and left in a jovial mood.

Monday 28 August 2006

The district nurse visited Mum today, as she does every Monday. Naturally, I had my ear to the door. When I confessed this to the nurse afterwards, she pointed out that she had deliberately spoken loudly for my benefit.

Anyway, it was not good news. Although Mum is keeping up a brave façade of happiness and reasonable health, she is really very insecure. She told the nurse how miserable she was when she was on her own, and that she's frightened of what will happen if I go back to Cape Town. Now that she can't paint any longer, life holds little for her. She's confined to the house because she's so weak, and now her reading ability is waning, too.

Clearly there's a lot more going on in Mum's head than I was aware of. She has all kinds of issues that are churning around inside her: will she have to go into a rest home; how miserable will she be there; will she die alone; how she will die; how much is she inconveniencing her children by dragging out her last days? I can see Mum feels she must plan her death, and because of her kind nature she is trying to do so without inconveniencing us. To do that means doing what to her is the unthinkable – going into a hospice or rest home. For other people, yes. For her, never.

The good news is that she looks healthy and is still smiling spontaneously and enjoying people's company. It is imperative that I arrange a continuous roster of family members staying with her. I'm still trying to coordinate with my siblings to come so that I can go back to Cape Town for a time. Originally, Fergus was prepared to be here by mid-

The Last Waltz: Love, Death & Betrayal

September, but now he is talking about late October. He speaks of the problem of getting leave from work and the difficulty in getting air tickets. He does acknowledge that the thought of being in Mum's house even for a couple of weeks with her in her present condition is too sad.

Mary certainly has a strong sense of responsibility towards Mum, and like me she struggles to get much time off from her work. So I have a problem.

The other complication in the timing of the visits is to make sure that Mary and Jo aren't here together. Their relationship over the years has been less than harmonious, and I don't want their life long feud boiling over beside mum's death bed, as Mum is searching to find her profound parting words to us.

Tuesday 29 August 2006

As soon as I get up in the mornings I open the curtain covering the French window in the lounge so that Mum can see from her bed (through the doorway of her room) the expansive and tranquil view. If I do it early enough, she can wake up to the view, but sometimes she beats me to it.

When I was boiling up my pot of vegetables for dinner, Mum came hovering around, waiting for me to drain them. She then drank the water as a soup, after she had added copious amounts of salt. I have seen her sprinkling salt on sweet things. Of course it is nonsense to suggest to her that she cut back now. She did say to me that I shouldn't get quite as addicted to salt as she is. I told her that was unlikely. As a non-smoker and social drinker, I obviously don't express these addictive personality genes.

Mum was curious to know why I drink so little alcohol. She speculates that it must be due to Dad's alcoholism. She said she thought that one of us might be affected by it. Maybe that was me. I was certainly aware of his drinking problem from an early age. Looking back, I am happier having had a father who was intoxicated on sherry rather than one intoxicated with himself.

I was a typical student boozer at university. And each trip home I did participate in Dad's drinking sessions, although

The Last Waltz: Love, Death & Betrayal

somewhat reluctantly. I remember after a meal he would bring out a selection of half a dozen liqueur bottles for us to sample. After a particular bottle was chosen, the men weren't allowed to leave the table until it was finished, while the women cleaned up in the kitchen. This was a variation of the older tradition of the men retiring to the drawing room for a cigar and port. The liqueur was not any cheap local one; it was usually imported Drambuie, Chartreuse or Benedictine.

The men usually consisted only of Dad, Jo's partner Roger, and me, so I certainly accounted for a good quarter of a bottle, much to Dad's pleasure. This was an unusual way of impressing one's father. The conventional approach would be with good study grades or sports achievements.

I recall one time that Dad was proud of me. It was when I wrote an article that appeared on the front page of the *Hokitika Guardian*. I described my life as a West Coast boy who had chosen to live in South Africa. One of the subheadings was "Chicken Run" under which I outlined how this expression was coined to describe the white South Africans who fled the country after the blacks took control of the government. Dad bought extra copies of this paper, circled the "Chicken Run" subheading, and then delivered one into the letterboxes of the four white South African doctors in Hokitika.

I do miss Dad's jovial dinner parties but I particularly miss Roger. He and Jo gave me hope for love and marriage. They met when she was nineteen and he was thirty-nine. He was very handsome, strong and rugged-looking, which negated the twenty years' age difference. Jo was stunningly beautiful and very feminine. They seemed to be a perfect match, always demonstrative in their affection for each other, and their relationship made me think that soul mates really do exist. I was shocked when I learnt a few years ago that they had broken up after being together for more than twenty years. They both still live in the isolated coastal region north of Greymouth, but they live separate lives apart from sharing their two sons. Orlando didn't suffer their separation as he had already left home, but I am sure Fabian was affected.

My ears are now totally blocked with earwax from the swimming. This has made my hikes up the hill especially peaceful – not only am I on my own here, but no sounds can intrude. It really is a bit like being in Tibet; solitude everywhere.

Thursday 31 August 2006

Today Mum was walking unassisted. I told her how much she was improving but she interrupted me: "I don't want to hear it." At lunch, Gwyneth asked me in front of Mum how long I would be staying. Again, Mum didn't want to hear it.

We bumped into an art friend Mum had not seen for a long time, and the first thing Mum told her is that she's got cancer. This is the second time I have heard her say this, and each time it's been a real conversation stopper. Later she told me she says this to put people at ease – so they know why she hasn't been at art classes, and why she looks so frail. I suggested in the future that she just tell them she hasn't been well.

We then did a bit of clothes shopping. Apparently, Mum threw out all her summer clothes some months ago as she thought she wouldn't need them. I think that, in buying the clothes, she's making a bold assumption: that summer will come to this part of the world.

Richard had said he would "Either" come for dinner tonight, "Or" if he couldn't get the kids, he'd come on Sunday. As it turned out he managed to get one of my nieces and a couple of friends. He brought food for my niece, as she seems to need a special teenage diet.

Friday 1 September 2006

Since I have been here, Mum has stopped me every time I've started to talk about the future, which includes her birthday. After the incident with Gwyneth yesterday, I decided to take things in hand. I insisted today that we talk about it.

First, I told her that we have to be realistic and assume that she'll be alive for her birthday, since it's just over a week away. With a sad sigh, she reluctantly agreed that this was the most likely scenario. All I needed to know was whether she wanted a birthday party or not, so that we could make the necessary arrangements. Mum hates to be the center of attention and a birthday dinner would force her into the limelight. She also dislikes having her house under scrutiny by lots of people. Mum has always lived in disorganized surroundings where only she knows where everything is, and to have to shape these surroundings into something presentable to a big gathering of friends was a little frightening for her.

I told her I needed to know her wishes, as I was sure something would be organized if I didn't nip it in the bud quickly. She was emphatic that there be no party – which I was disappointed about – just a family dinner at Richard's place on Crosby Street. She said that she always has her birthday dinners there. I'll talk to Richard.

I then told her she had to be prepared for my returning to Cape Town for a few weeks, and that I was negotiating with the others to have them all come and stay in overlapping sequence so that she wouldn't be alone. I said that maybe there'd be one gap of a week, and that Richard had suggested Jonah stay with her then. She's at a loose end at present. Mum was unsettled by this suggestion. Richard had also proposed that his daughters stay that week, but again Mum was not taken by the idea. I said we could keep exploring the possibility of a rest home for that period.

At least she's facing up to the fact that she's not going to drop dead immediately. She is ruefully mourning the fact that she could well live to Christmas and beyond. She said she can't understand, when she's so riddled with cancer, why she's been feeling so healthy.

I told her that if the world starts falling apart I will make sure I am back in Dunedin, because the safest place to be reading about it will be here in the *Otago Daily Times*.

Sunday 3 September 2006

We had an unscheduled outing today. We were invited to join Richard for Father's Day lunch at a restaurant where one of his daughters works on the weekends.

The Last Waltz: Love, Death & Betrayal

Richard phoned in the morning to say that the restaurant was fully booked. He said that Mum and I should go nevertheless. He would "Either" meet us there, he said, "Or", if he could get a booking at an alternative place, he would let me know by cell phone. His daughter, who was working there today, phoned to tell him we shouldn't come – there was a long waiting list for tables. But he wanted to try on the off chance. Richard's not good when it comes to organizing events and people, and it's ironic because it's his favorite pastime. He must have driven Mary crazy, seeing she's completely the opposite. This seems to me like a reasonable basis for divorce!

Richard arrived with Elizabeth Ellis – a new friend in his wide social circle – and they came and greeted Mum who was waiting in the car. I explained about the restaurant being overbooked and suggested we go elsewhere for lunch. To this Elizabeth replied, "Not at all," and assured us that we'd have a table very soon, on the grounds that she knew the owner of "this establishment." She then went gliding off into the restaurant and straight up the stairs to his office. And sure enough, we were seated within ten minutes. It was impressive, and also a little awkward, breezing past the queue of patient patrons.

Lunch was pleasant, with a group of about ten of us. I kept Mum company with a bowl of soup. Elizabeth sat on the other side of her, and was superb in the way she coordinated the conversation at the table and did all the hard work. She must be about sixty and she comes across as a glamorous, self-assured, and diplomatic social butterfly. I don't know the background to her elevated social status. Surprisingly, she isn't forceful or bossy.

Everyone decided to come to Mum's for coffee after lunch. Elizabeth loved the idea as she seemed drawn to Mum and was keen to see her house. Mum, by contrast, was very anxious that her house wouldn't match up to Elizabeth's high-society standards. If this were the case, though, Elizabeth's the sort of person who would be too well bred to show it.

While the others had pudding, Mum and I charged back to her place, to get a head start on the necessary preparations.

The Last Waltz: Love, Death & Betrayal

Mum's never been particular about the tidiness of her house; things tend to be where they are most convenient. I've noticed this especially when I've travelled with her. Each destination, whether one night or many, she would open her suitcase and give it a little flick. Things would fall out and stay where they landed until they were either used or packed away when we moved on.

Throughout her life she only dusted or used a vacuum cleaner in the frantic moments before she was expecting visitors. I remember that Dad, who was much more fastidious about cleaning, used to unsubtly leave the vacuum cleaner at her feet when she was in her normal relaxing position of reading books with her feet up and listening to her Bach records, and hope she got the hint. I can't remember if Dad ever did any vacuuming himself.

Now Mum lives in her charming rustic cottage, hidden away from the world, and she does what she wants. The cupboards and fridge are always cluttered and full of jars and bottles of sauces and jams that are way past their expiry date.

With her artistic streak, Mum's house is full of unusual ornaments that were made by her, given by friends, or collected in her travels around the world. In addition, she has been a lifelong collector of antiques, both furniture and crockery. The combination of antiquities and Mum's disorganization leads to a home with a comfortable feel about it. You can relax and know that you can do whatever you like without disturbing the harmony. However, since we kids are generally tidier than she is, the net result of our visits is an overall improvement in the tidiness of the house.

So today, with the visitors coming, led by the glamorous Elizabeth Ellis, we managed to squeeze in an hour of intensive cleaning before they arrived. Mum was fairly mobile – and pragmatic. She used the stove and the fridge and the sink for support while she cleaned them. It was impressive to see how a visit from Elizabeth mustered the resolve in Mum to clean up.

I did the vacuuming and straightening of carpets, and put away the newspapers, books and photo albums.

Elizabeth seemed suitably impressed when she arrived for her inspection of the premises. We had coffee and biscuits and it was all very sociable. She left full of promises and plans to stay in touch with Mum.

Inviting Elizabeth into her house was certainly Mum's excitement for the day, something different for her from her normal routine. I then went for a hike to Larnach's Castle to let today's drama ebb away.

Monday 4 September 2006

It was a gloriously sunny day here, which helped to keep my spirits up. Apart from that I felt a bit miserable that Mum's world is now so limited. Most of her time is spent in bed listening to radio interviews, reading, or doing the crosswords. I try to see to it that each day has a focus or highlight. There is almost always a visitor – one of the local artists or retired doctors. Other days the highlight might be a TV program – a BBC documentary or drama.

The district nurse came to see Mum today. I listened at the door as well and heard Mum say that having me there gave her a reason to live. It cheered me up.

Since it was such a nice day Mum took me on a slow tour outside. She has always loved creating wild and natural-looking gardens. It has been easy while living alone in Dunedin, but while Dad was alive it was a tricky undertaking for her to do any gardening. Dad was always stopping her with his booming voice when he caught her doing anything even slightly creative in the garden. It got to the point where she used to get up before him in the morning to sneak around the garden doing all the things that were banned. One of her main goals was to keep extending the boundary of her various flowerbeds and rock gardens. She did this with a piecemeal approach, extending each garden a few inches at a time so Dad wouldn't notice. By the time he surfaced in the mornings she would be in her book-reading posture on the couch, looking completely innocent.

In spite of this intense surveillance of the garden, both Mum and Dad failed to notice that as a joke Fergus had planted some marijuana seeds in the rock garden in the middle of the back lawn. These had grown strong healthy stems by the time Christmas came around. Every Christmas

The Last Waltz: Love, Death & Betrayal

Dad would host the local dignitaries to a small Christmas lunchtime party. This involved the local police sergeant who quietly pointed out to Mum that she had a fine crop in her garden. Mum went on a quick search and destroy mission before Dad found out.

"Before Dad finds out." This phrase encapsulates so much of those days. Dad was a difficult man to live with. As kids, Jo and I often discussed why Mum stayed with him when he was so domineering. I think a lot of women define themselves by the man they are with. They don't feel whole unless they are in a relationship even if it is a bad one. They don't know that it is okay to be alone. When Mum eventually found herself alone when Dad died, I didn't think it would affect her too badly and that her creative spirit would blossom with the new freedom she had gained. But this was not the case. It took her a good two years to get used to the solitude. She spent most of that time in the granny cabin, painting landscapes. She told me that she couldn't stand being alone in a house that was once so full of Dad's presence. He had dominated her so much that she found it hard to deal with the total freedom of being able to do what she liked when she liked. No longer did she have to sneak around the garden before he woke in the morning. No longer did she have to plan her afternoon around having dinner on the table at exactly seven, or face his fury. No longer was her existence defined by Dad. Without him, for a while, it was as if she didn't exist.

Today I met Jim, my Ph.D. supervisor, for lunch. He successfully twisted my arm into giving a seminar to the Microbiology Department. I told him I wanted to do it soon, before Mum's health deteriorated. I chatted to Ian on the phone tonight. He invited me to stay at his place for a few nights if I needed to get some rest from looking after Mum. I asked him if he still snored, and he said he did. I said I would get more rest sleeping at the railway station slope. I asked how Sandra coped with his snoring, and he said she uses industrial-strength earplugs. She can still hear him.

The Last Waltz: Love, Death & Betrayal

Tuesday 5 September 2006

Mum fell over in the middle of the night while getting up to go to the toilet. Even from my room I heard this because I've been sleeping so lightly. She didn't hurt herself and she put the fall down to tripping on a book on the floor.

I had a good swim today, followed by coffee at the Italian café. I'm glad I haven't picked up a cold or cough yet. If I passed a bad cold on to Mum it could kill her, although somehow I think she might appreciate that. What I *have* picked up is lots of itchy bites. I hope it's the odd flea on Truffle and not no-see-ums on the mattress. I've just finished giving all of my bedding a wash and an airing.

Mum is eating reasonably well. She now has a small plate of whatever I'm cooking, and tonight she really enjoyed the mackerel and pasta. I'll keep making it to encourage her to eat, and at the moment I'm making sure there's a constant supply of bread-and--butter pudding. She heats up a little of this each night in the oven and covers it with cream liqueur and a small spoon of ice cream. This is good news, considering that she was only drinking soup when I got here.

Tonight Mum was reading the book Alex had sent her for her birthday two years ago, *Wild Swans: Three Daughters of China*, by Jung Chang. Inside Alex had written: "Dear Mama Davison, this book is about intelligent, courageous, and caring women. I loved it, and it reminded me of you." Mum stopped reading and commented on how wonderful it was that Alex and I had stayed such good friends when we had broken up so many years ago. I think Mum is more concerned that I have children than that I have a love match for life. She thinks children are more important in providing happiness and security.

I don't have any doubts whatsoever that I want kids. I have always looked forward to the day of being a father. Children bring a lot of pleasure to your life, and until now I have had to direct this paternal energy towards Cleo and Caesar. It is not only the pleasure children bring, but they also represent a configuration of one's own self. They carry your genes, and your family ancestry and values. They are the most significant monuments that you leave behind in this life.

Wednesday 6 September 2006

Mum is now almost totally bald with only a tuft of fringe sticking out at the front of her beanie. It's all disappeared in the last two weeks. It must be distressing for her, and I can't say I enjoy this either. She keeps her head covered with the woolen hats she's been knitting for herself and she's at great pains not to let me see that she is bald. This is out of her control, as while she's sleeping her hat has usually worked its way off by the time I come in to see her in the mornings. I put it back on in the same motion of waking her, so that she doesn't have to know.

I am bombarded by little shocks each day as I watch Mum dying before my eyes. I pound up and down the length of the pool to temporarily free my mind of the pain of them. Today I went for a two-hour hike instead of a swim while Doug was visiting. When I got back I overheard him saying he had to go now, as his wife was expecting him to come and help prepare the dinner. He said this three times before he eventually left, forty-five minutes later. He must have an understanding wife.

Tonight Mum discovered that rice pudding is not so bad after all, when covered with cream liqueur. She previously said she was not keen to try it. I told her how it was just as important to say when you don't like something that is cooked for you, as it is to compliment something you do enjoy. I told her about my Cape Town bridge evenings at Richard and Helen's, where I pretended that Helen's nougat was delicious. I really hate nougat, but after I politely said how much I enjoyed it the first time it became a regular treat. At this point Mum meekly said, "You know that mackerel dish you cooked last night which I said was so nice? I didn't want to tell you this, but in truth, I really don't like mackerel."

The Last Waltz: Love, Death & Betrayal

Thursday 7 September 2006

Today's shock was the biggest so far. Thursday is our weekly trip to town and lunch with Gwyneth, and after lunch Mum wanted to stop in at the Otago Art Society gallery, situated on the main highway out of Dunedin. She often goes – or rather used to go – to see an artist's work or a particular painting. When we got there, I helped her out of the car and went back to lock my door, leaving her to start on her way to the gallery because she likes this illusion of her independence. It was noisy with traffic and I had my back to the pavement. When I turned, I saw her sprawled at the side of the road, with blood on her face, and scrambling for her hat.

Amidst the chaos she was calling out, "My hat, my hat!"

It turned out she was unharmed. The blood was a minor scratch, but she must have got a bad knock on the head. I got her up on her feet, wiped off the blood, and, with her hat firmly back on, she trotted off into the art gallery as if nothing had happened. A group of nurses who had witnessed the fall came rushing over to ask me if I realized that she had received a big bang on the head, but I tried to play the episode down. Mum is from quite a different generation, the wartime generation. People seemed emotionally stronger in those days and typically rose above disappointments and tragedy with humor and resolve.

Tonight Mum has her feet up, listening to music. She's losing the ability to read easily; she finds she has to read slowly to concentrate on the story. I asked her if she had a headache from today's fall and she said, after thinking about it carefully, that she did have a slight one, but probably only because I had drawn her attention to it. She said, "I'm sure if you hadn't mentioned it, I wouldn't have one," then added, "I suspect everyone has a headache if they think hard enough about it. Have you got a headache?"

I thought about this and replied, "Yes, I think I probably have."

I loved this attempt at playing down the effect of her dramatic fall, although I think today's events were more of a shock for me than for her. Anything that Mum does out of the ordinary she explains away in rational terms. If I had asked her why she fell over today, she probably would have blamed a pothole in the road. But I feel this is the beginning of a pattern. And it was certainly quite a dramatic way for Mum to demonstrate that this pattern may have begun.

I'm now going to cook up something to tempt her appetite. Not mackerel and pasta.

Friday 8 September 2006

I see a few daffodils have broken out from underground around Dunedin. They have probably finished flowering in Cape Town. The days are getting longer by three and a half minutes. By Christmas time there will still be daylight at bedtime. I wonder where I will be for Christmas.

Mum gets up each afternoon at one and then goes back to bed at seven. During this time "up" she spends most of the afternoon lying on her bed listening to the radio, or reading. When I suggested to her that she may as well stay in bed all day and save the hassle of getting up and dressed, she said that the main reason she got up at all was to have the pleasure of going back to bed later.

I am keeping things quiet for her today after yesterday's drama. My lecture is coming up on Monday, which I'm dreading. The prospect of lecturing to all of my old professors is stressful. I see that they have put posters up to announce it as a "keynote lecture."

I'm now off to buy old ladies' nighties. Mum has given me very specific instructions on what type of nighty she wants and where to get them. The most important thing is that they are pure cotton. Secondly, they must be large or extra-large, as she really likes to swim in them.

Saturday 9 September 2006

I made Mum's birthday cake tonight. She heard me knocking around in the kitchen and couldn't resist coming to see what I was up to. She loves to be there to see what I am doing, although I imagine it is just the social interaction she craves. This is a role reversal from when I was a boy and always wanted to be a part of the action whenever Mum was making a cake. In my case I think the licking of the bowl was the great attraction. This childhood pleasure was destroyed when Mum added a rubber scraper to her baking utensils.

Mum understands the importance of giving a talk to my old department on her birthday. Again, it's another case of bad timing.

Monday 11 September 2006

First thing I did this morning was congratulate Mum on making it to eighty-five, the same age that her mother died, and one year older than Great-Aunt Edith, her mother's sister. She's very similar to them both. She inherited her mother's mathematical brain and her aunt's love of travelling.

The last trip I shared with Mum was to Kathmandu at the base of the Himalayas. This was to commemorate the year in which she turned eighty, and Fergus and I fifty and forty respectively. The conditions in Nepal were very testing for her because of the heat and the dust and the risks of food poisoning. She was the only one who didn't get sick.

Over coffee we joked about how certain she was when I arrived that she wouldn't be here for her birthday. In keeping with this expectation, I hadn't brought a present with me from South Africa. I suggested that she could well now make it into next year but her reply, as usual, was that she didn't want to talk about it. In lieu of a present I gave her a selection of sweets from Dunedin, and she particularly liked the Russian fudge. Of course I didn't talk about my plans to go back to Cape Town, but the thought was in the air, and I could see how sad it makes her. She would be so content to pass the hours of her last days in the companionable routine of my bringing her coffee each morning, chatting to her on and off through the day while I work from my room and then sitting down to watch our usual programs in the evening. I would also love to do this, but in terms of my own life it just doesn't make sense. I could end up being here for another six months . . . or more?

The Last Waltz: Love, Death & Betrayal

I sat with Mum during the morning and coordinated a few phone calls from friends and family members. She was delighted by the first call from Bebe in Cape Town. They have been close friends in spite of the distance between them. It is wonderful how they express their friendship through the exchange of recipes.

Later in the morning I gave her the cake I'd made. It had the traditional arrangement of one candle to mark each decade plus one for each single year, making a total of thirteen candles. She made a wish, and blew them out without any difficulty. I suspect her wish was for a quick and painless death by heart attack. She really has pinned all her hopes on this.

I gave my seminar on DNA forensics, which I linked to the September 11 terrorist attacks, to match today's anniversary of the event. Norton arrived in the middle of it and took up a seat near the front. I took the opportunity to make a semi-serious remark about how his research team's patenting of the human genome for use in human DNA identifications more than twenty years ago restricts my own research. Norton just loved the attention, and took up the gauntlet. He fired a few questions at me throughout the rest of my talk and these served to highlight the relevance of my research. I couldn't have stage-managed it better, and I owe him a bagful of muesli bars.

After the talk I picked up a cake at the supermarket and a big supply of candles. Richard had roasted lamb for dinner and at the table were Mum and me from Broad Bay, Richard and my nieces from Crosby Street, plus four of Richard's friends who all knew Mum, including Jonah. At Mum's request this dinner was meant to be only family, and it was quite an effort on my part to stop Richard from inviting more, but Mum seemed more than happy with these extra faces, although she did seem very tired. A large group at the table helped to keep the atmosphere light and cheerful. After dinner we had a sponge with eighty-five candles, and with impressive lung capacity, Mum blew them all out in one go. The candles generated so much heat that they destroyed the sponge on top. Luckily it was there just for show and there was a nicer cake underneath it, which the teenagers devoured. I made a brief video of the evening.

I stayed up after midnight watching TV with Mum. She watched from her bed and knitted. When I said goodnight she said how happy she was having me stay up late with her for company. I realize now that I should change my clock and stay up until after she has bathed and gone to bed, rather than disappearing early and leaving her to negotiate the bathroom and house alone. Originally, it was a strategy to give her some privacy for bathing.

One thing that worries me is that she has stopped bathing every night. I am concerned only because, all her life, a bath a day has been an absolute matter of principle for her. No matter where we've been in the world, she'd always tracked one down. But now I see she is struggling with her bathing routine. It must be exhausting for her to get in and out, and it makes sense for me to at least be on hand in case she should need help. At the same time, I know she'd be mortified if she did.

Anyway, I can see that she's still quite happy, which is extraordinary under the circumstances.

Tuesday 12 September 2006

Another friend of Mum's wanted to drop by, but I told her it wasn't a good day to visit. For the first time, Mum admitted she isn't always happy to have visitors. She has to try to concentrate on what they say until she pretends to be asleep. Mum has reached a stage where she prefers my company because I fit easily into her daily routine without causing any stress. Now that she has me, she is not feeling the same need for her daily visitors.

Mum asked me if it was all right if she didn't bath again, two nights in a row. She was almost apologetic, but I assured her that she didn't smell, and that most of the population of England bath only once a week, so it is said.

The Last Waltz: Love, Death & Betrayal

Thursday 14 September 2006

Today being Thursday, once again we drove into town for lunch with Gwyneth. I could see that Mum was noticeably weaker. When I dropped her off at the restaurant in the Octagon, she couldn't walk without leaning on me, and when I picked her up after playing tennis she wanted me to bring the car up to outside the restaurant, rather than walk the short distance to where the car was parked. In one way she seemed embarrassed by her request, but she also had a cheeky smile as if to say, "It's hard to believe but it's true." We then stopped off at the supermarket and I did a quick shop while she waited in the car.

Friday 15 September 2006

It is midnight and I'm having a dramatic night with Mum.

The day had seemed fairly ordinary. Doug came to visit in the afternoon and I drove to Dunedin for a swim. He was still here when I got back two hours later and was chatting happily with Mum. After he'd gone, I cooked dinner and Mum heated up a tin of chicken soup for herself. I think she drank only half a cup of this, and I can't remember her drinking much during the day. She went to bed early, feeling very tired. When I checked on her before I went to bed, she said she felt like being sick. She asked me to bring her a bowl and as soon as I did she started vomiting into it.

I stayed up watching TV so that I could monitor her condition, and later she asked me to escort her to the toilet because she was feeling so weak and nauseous. On the way back she could hardly stand up, and even with my support kept stumbling. She then dropped to the floor on her hands and knees so she could vomit. In the process her hat came off.

I felt such pity and such love. My once dignified and elegant mother reduced to this. I also fully realized at this moment that there was only one direction her health could take from here. It was only going to get worse.

The Last Waltz: Love, Death & Betrayal

I am now going to sleep with my ear alert to Mum's call in case she needs to go to the bathroom again. It could be a disrupted night ahead.

Saturday 16 September 2006

Mum is now in hospital on a drip after being taken there by ambulance this morning. I had checked on her a few times during the night. She vomited only once more, and felt better afterwards, but when I awoke in the morning she seemed barely conscious. She was able to listen to me and respond with a weak voice. I offered her drinks of Marmite and water, which she had small sips of. As the morning progressed, she was showing no improvement and I was at a loss for what to do. I knew Mum just hated anyone making a fuss over her when she was sick and I didn't think I could phone her doctor without her approval, so I didn't even ask. I knew she was too weak to get into the car. This was a situation I had never been in and I was reluctant to take control and tell my mother what to do when it had always been her who decided everything concerning her own health, and she'd never liked being told anything by other people in this respect.

Here I was observing her in a state where she was not really fit to gauge her own health and what action should be taken, and I was feeling powerless to do anything for fear of treading on what was clearly her turf. As the morning progressed, I finally plucked up the courage and asked her if she would mind if I phoned Dr. MacDonald for his advice. I was really surprised when she immediately nodded her head and said I could.

I was unable to get hold of Dr. MacDonald but left a message for him to call me. I then reluctantly left Mum and went to the airport, where I had previously arranged to meet a friend. On the way Dr. MacDonald phoned me back and I explained what had happened last night and how Mum was now very weak. He said she must get to hospital immediately and he would arrange for an ambulance. I then phoned Mum from my cell phone to tell her the arrangement, fearing what her reaction to this would be. Fortunately she had already spoken to Dr. MacDonald, and seemed quite relaxed. I then

The Last Waltz: Love, Death & Betrayal

got another call from Dr. MacDonald to tell me an ambulance would be there at twelve, by which time I would be back from the airport.

I was back before the ambulance got to Mum's place and was able to calm any anxiety she might have about being taken to hospital. As it turned out, she was quite relaxed and told me she had a bag under the bed containing all she needed for her stay. Perhaps this is what she has always wanted.

The ambulance arrived and the paramedics loaded Mum on a stretcher and into the back. I joked with Mum and told her that she was going to have an exciting ride and asked if they would be sounding the siren. The nurse replied that when an ambulance siren sounded it was a certain indication that the person inside would not be enjoying the ride. I was silenced.

I followed it to the hospital in a state of anxiety. When I arrived at the Accident & Emergency reception, the receptionist asked me to confirm the personal details of my mother. The first question she asked was, "Was your mother born in Istanbul, Turkey?"

Istanbul Turkey, Istanbul Turkey, the words just rang in my ears.

Of course I knew she was born in Istanbul, Turkey (or Constantinople, as she preferred). But in that moment of being reminded of that fact, my mother's extraordinary past flashed through my mind. For so many weeks I had been so absorbed in watching her failing health, meeting her friends, and focusing on her recent artist's life in Broad Bay, that her extraordinary past was forgotten.

I wanted to see Mum as soon as possible. When I was allowed in I found her on a bed in a separate room in the ward. She still hadn't been seen by a doctor. I was sure she would be very upset at having to come to hospital but she looked more at peace than I had seen her for a long time. She spoke calmly and even joked about some things she had seen in the ward while she was waiting. She has said to me several times in long-distance telephone conversations that she found it difficult to be her own doctor. Because she lived alone it was not easy for her to assess the day-to-day changes in her health. She had been her own doctor all her life and the time had come to let go of this role. Perhaps she was seeing an opportunity to do this now that she was in hospital surrounded by medical experts.

I stayed with her for an hour or so and said I would return later in the afternoon after she had been examined, to see what the diagnosis is. I also promised to bring her some Mogadons, as she feared she might be denied these as had happened on her previous stay for her colonoscopy operation. Apparently the new generation of doctors and nurses are opposed to Mogadon because it has a long half-life and is very habit-forming. Mum has been taking them every night for many years without any side effects and could see no reason to change now.

In the evening Mum was on a drip in a room shared with three other elderly ladies. She was looking even more tranquil. Her blood test results had come through and they indicated that she had been suffering from dehydration and that this had caused her vomiting and falling into a semiconscious state this morning.

I am hardly surprised that she was dehydrated as she doesn't eat or drink very much at the best of times. I think yesterday she unwittingly drank less than she usually does. Now that she is on a drip her demeanor has picked up a lot.

She didn't want anything else to eat or drink as the drip seems to keep everything in balance. I put a few Mogadon tablets inside the sock on her right foot in case the nursing staff wouldn't give her any. Mum loved this act of defiance!

I gave her a hug and said I would phone in the morning to see if she wanted me to bring anything. She hadn't seen a specialist doctor yet and I told her that I would like to be there when she did. I wondered how she was going to feel about this young hospital staff giving her baths and taking her to the toilet. I am sure she was dreading the thought.

I am off for an early night now as I am exhausted after the drama of last night and today's anxiety.

At least tonight I can lock the door for the first time. Having spent fifteen years in Cape Town where we lock ourselves into prisons at night, with burglar bars on every window, security gates on every door and alarms attached to every door and opening window, it has been hard to adjust to Mum's sleeping with the door open most nights so that Truffle can come and go as she pleases.

I'm sorry, Truffle, but things are going to be a little different with me in charge.

Sunday 17 September 2006

I phoned Mum in the morning and got a list of what she wanted: slippers, nighties, hand mirror, knitted hat and Campbell's tinned chicken soup.

When I got to the hospital it took me a while to find her as she had been moved to a different ward where she had a room to herself with a view overlooking the city. Norton was sitting by her bedside telling her stories when I got there. He had phoned me yesterday to arrange his usual weekend visit but on hearing that Mum was in hospital he rescheduled his weekend to deliver the muesli bar to her here.

Norton is quite a ladies' man and was quick to tell me how he had had the honor of accompanying Mum to her new room, and then present her with a muesli bar. I think it's wonderful that Mum should have such male admirers at age eighty-five. As soon as Norton left she quickly gave his muesli bar to me and asked me to eat it. I told her I didn't eat food that came unwrapped and was hand delivered! She then asked me to take it with me so as not to offend Norton when he next visited.

Mum was feeling much better now that she had rehydrated, but her big fear was that she might be discharged today. I also thought it possible as I couldn't think why they would keep her when she was now stable. I was pleased that she was happy being in hospital; it was a good practice run, in case she had to come in again, or stay in a hospice or rest home. Mum was very content having people running around looking after her. She didn't eat any of the hospital lunch that arrived while I was there. She seemed to think the drip was enough to keep her nourished.

A nurse came and asked if she would like a shower, and Mum, who has probably never showered in her life, gave a big smile and said, "Yes, please." It was a pleasing revelation that Mum was willing to be showered by a stranger.

I left for my daily swim and came back late in the afternoon. Mum had still not been seen by a doctor. I found out that this would not happen until Monday and that she would be kept in at least until then. The nurse indicated that Mum would not be discharged until she was drinking liquids on her own. I told her this and she seemed relieved; she was really taking to the idea of being in hospital. I decided I'd better organize some visitors soon as this is what she enjoys most about hospitals.

Tonight I had a drink with Ian near the hospital. Like worn-out gramophone records, we always end up rehashing all the hilarious stories from our student days.

We have known each other for twenty-five years and our friendship has never faltered. We have totally different backgrounds, and for that matter, futures. I often speculate on how I befriended him so easily and have not found a similar friend on my travels. It had to be more than shared interests: sport is hardly the cement for a life-long bond. I think perhaps it is our shared secrets. As students we told each other our innermost fears, weaknesses, and dreams. Things I'm sure neither of us told to anyone else. On top of that we shared the same disappointments and joys of those difficult years growing up in our early twenties. I would trust Ian with my life, as he would me.

After drinks I managed to get past the hospital security system after visiting hours, and crept into Mum's room to give her a goodnight hug. She was awake listening to the radio when I got there. She had had no more visitors, which was hardly surprising since not many people knew she was in hospital. Richard had phoned and said "Either" he would come in the afternoon "Or" later in the evening. As the hospital doors were now locked it was obvious that neither the "Either" nor the "Or" would happen. I told her to have an early night as the hospital nurses were sure to wake her at dawn.

I have been keeping my siblings up to speed on the state of Mum's health. It probably sounds worse than it is, but if I were still in Cape Town I would be on a plane by now. Jo and Mary are both planning to make visits in the very near future. Fergus is going to sit tight and wait for instructions.

Monday 18 September 2006

I sat with Mum for a couple of hours this morning. It is quite entertaining watching the staff coming in and out, treating Mum like a child, and Mum giving me that little knowing glance each time as if to say, "Isn't this funny. They don't know they are dealing with a doctor." She also makes a great joke of how it is a different nurse who sees her each time, none of them seeming to know why she is there and when she will be discharged. Mum feels she hasn't seen a doctor until she has seen the consultant oncologist.

I left for a swim when a group of Mum's lady art friends came to visit her. It is quite something to behold the way these "arty ladies" bond so well with each other, when the only thing they initially had in common was a desire to paint. Until recently, Mum didn't want them to know her age because they are all a good ten to twenty years younger. I was surprised that people of Mum's age would care a damn about it. Was she embarrassed to be so much older, or did she think that they would think she was too old to befriend? I wonder if Mum can now see how these people almost worship her.

I have gotten to know these artists through their paintings and the many funny stories coming out of their classes. The most recent one I heard was when they painted nude models, and at one Saturday morning class the model did not turn up, so rather than cancel the class, one of the artists stripped off her clothes and posed for the others. In Cape Town I have so many of Mum's nude paintings I am thinking of wallpapering my bedroom with them.

When I came back to the hospital in the afternoon, Gwyneth was visiting but was just on her way out. Gwyneth tends to be much disciplined in staying for only one hour for each person she visits.

I was enjoying myself as much as Mum today with all of these interesting characters popping in and out among the

The Last Waltz: Love, Death & Betrayal

hospital staff. Mum continued her running commentary about what the staff was doing and how unnecessary it was.

The next cast member to enter from stage left was none other than Dr. MacDonald. Mum was genuinely very happy to see him. Finally a medical person she could confide in and trust had arrived. Although Mum was Dr. MacDonald's private patient, her treatment in the hospital was out of his control. Also he was not a specialist in oncology and therefore not able to throw much light on the current status of her health. Mum gave her standard speech to Dr. MacDonald about not wanting her misery to continue and wanting to die soon. Dr. MacDonald gave his standard reply that she didn't have long to go. Such words were music to Mum's ears; he had only to say them every time he saw her.

Dr. MacDonald wanted to speak with me in private outside her room. He didn't really have much to say that required this secrecy but essentially repeated what he had said in his office shortly after I arrived, that Mum didn't have long to go and I should tell my siblings that they should come now if they wanted to say goodbye to her. He is such a kind and gentle man, I could understand why Mum is so happy to have him as her private doctor.

I wanted to ask him if he could give Mum something to speed up her exit from this world when it became unbearable. But I knew that such a question would be unfair because euthanasia is illegal in New Zealand. I cannot blame him or other doctors for not helping someone who wants to die. They have sworn allegiance to the Hippocratic Oath, the rite of passage for practitioners of medicine. It is almost a religious oath that most tend to follow without question.

There is one defining line: "I will prescribe regimens for the good of my patients according to my ability and my judgment and never do harm to anyone."

For the good of their patients? And what if their patients are old and want to die, is it really doing good not to help them?

When I returned to Mum's room she was anxious to know what Dr. MacDonald and I were talking about behind her back, yet at the same time pleased that by so doing we were indicating that we were taking the doctoring away from her.

The Last Waltz: Love, Death & Betrayal

I went out and had dinner at a Chinese restaurant around the corner. When I came back Jonah was sitting there with Mum. Mum was pleased to see me as she wanted her chicken soup and she wasn't confident Jonah would get it right. She indicated to me that she wanted Jonah to leave. I discreetly edged her out, implying that I wanted to be alone with Mum.

Once Jonah had left, Mum asked me to water a very thirsty-looking pot plant that one of her visitors had given her. I filled a glass and was about to do so when she said, "Make sure you pour it into the center of the plant at the base."

Grrrr... I have been watering my own pot plants for over twenty years, but I bit my tongue.

Instead, I told her that I have started seeing the students in my classes as my garden plants. It is very dry in Cape Town and it is a constant struggle for plants to survive. I give the weakest ones the greatest amount of attention and water, but eventually I come to the point where I decide to economize on resources and focus on those who have adapted well and leave the strugglers to the forces of natural selection.

Mum said, "That's extraordinary. I have always seen my patients as pot plants, but don't tell anyone that."

For us both to independently form this analogy is an example of "memes." These are inherited personality traits and ways of thinking. Memes are very hard to document scientifically, but are plainly obvious in families. Often parents and children have similar personalities, mannerisms and ways of thinking, even if they have had no contact with each other.

I remember when Mum visited Cape Town and she reprimanded me for showing scant regard for authority. Later that week we were on top of Table Mountain and I saw her climbing over a small fence with a "do not enter" sign, to study an unusual species of plant.

Tuesday 19 September 2006

Since I am not a morning person I didn't go to the hospital before 10am. By this time quite a lot has happened in Mum's day. Today I learnt that Richard had visited earlier in the morning as the "Either" had worked out before the "Or" had become necessary. Mum said he stood around for about ten minutes looking very awkward and not knowing quite what to say, and then disappeared because he had an important engagement to go to. Poor Richard. I can just imagine him standing at the end of the bed, fidgeting with his tie and glancing at his watch and wondering how early he could escape without being rude, probably discussing with Mum the cost of hospital care in New Zealand. At least as a lawyer he is expected to have important appointments to rush off to, and of course Mum knows Richard so well she has no reason to be offended. She really appreciates all that Richard has done for her. Even if he can't express his emotions, his actions indicate that he helps her from his heart rather than out of duty.

Shortly after I arrived the nurse came in and told me that Mum had had a fall during the night when she attempted to go to the toilet unassisted. She condescendingly called Mum a "bad girl" for not ringing the bell as she had been told. When the nurse left I scolded Mum and said, "You mustn't be a bad girl any more." Whatever the reason, Mum still had had a fall and I need to be aware of this potential when she comes home. Mum keeps hinting at the fact that she wants to stay longer in hospital.

Today I took a big pile of marking to the hospital and set up a mini-office in Mum's room with my table looking out the window over the city. Marking doesn't take intense concentration so I wasn't distracted by hospital staff popping in during the day.

The most significant of these was the specialist oncologist. I left him alone while he examined Mum. Afterwards he spoke to me in confidence outside the room. He said she was improving and would soon be back to how she had been, and that, with the best treatments available, she had some good quality life ahead of her.

After he continued on his rounds I was left to ponder why doctors insist on prolonging the inevitable. There is no treatment or medication for death.

Why do they assume it is a self-evident truth that avoidance of death is a good thing?

The Last Waltz: Love, Death & Betrayal

Some people choose to die and there is no reason to fear this.

The afternoon was very quiet with no visitors. Mum was listening to her radio with the earphones and her eyes closed, possibly asleep. At one point I turned around and stared at her and I concentrated my mind, thinking to myself, "Open your eyes, Mum, open your eyes."

Not surprisingly nothing happened, but the moment I turned my back on her to continue my marking she said, "Did you say something to me?"

I told her what I had just been thinking, and we were in agreement that this had been mental telepathy. Neither of us was particularly surprised by this as we have always been believers in it. Even though we are both scientists, we are broadminded enough to realize that there is a lot about life that is not understood and cannot be explained by science. Mum described what had happened as a "Sheldrake experience."

Rupert Sheldrake is one of our favorite science writers. His main theory is that all life is linked by invisible connections he calls morphogenetic fields. These are invisible fields such as you get between two magnets that repel each other. Some of his theories he tested scientifically and proved to be correct beyond statistical probability: testing to see if blindfolded amputees knew when their phantom limb was being touched; cats and dogs getting excited when their master left work to come home; homing pigeons being able to find their home even if it had been moved.

When I was a university student Mum and I talked a lot about the paranormal and we decided to form a death-communication pact, whereby the first one to die would make an attempt to communicate with the other one. Presumably Mum would die first, and I told her not to try to communicate with me if it meant that she was going to be "left behind" from whatever was waiting for her after death. I feared that this is where poltergeists come from! I suggested the best means of communication could be through an object closely associated with her, such as a pottery item that she had made. I also said that, if it were the only way, she should communicate with me in a dream, but this was a last resort as I would be bound to dream about her anyway after she died. Although Mum was broadminded about the many things science could not explain, she was very definite about what awaited people after death. She has always been certain that death is the end, and for that reason was convinced that our pact could come to nothing. I have reminded her of it several times since I have been back, as the time to put it to the test is near.

I went for a swim and a Chinese takeaway. When I came back Jonah was on her way out. She told me she had left a present for Mum and me. It was a small peppermint tin. Inside it was a good-sized ball of marijuana. Mum asked me to take it with me and not leave it lying around her room.

Mum and I then talked for a couple of hours. There was something surreal about the atmosphere in the hospital tonight. It was almost dreamlike the way Mum and I talked about death. It was as if we were not really there and were communicating from our subconscious. The room and corridor lights were very dim. There was no background noise as the patients were asleep. I mostly sat on the side of her bed as I do at home. We talked a lot about her desire to end her life before her brain deteriorated and she had no self-awareness. Taking her own life has become a constant theme of our discussions. She said her life now was too unpleasant, she felt uncomfortable all the time and had no desire to eat, and what she did eat had the same unpalatable taste. But the overriding point was that her death was near, so why shouldn't she just take that final step to finish it? She said she would no longer eat any solid food at all to give her more control of her death.

When I left tonight we had a long cheek-to-cheek hug. She said, "You are such a wonderful son." Mum had never said this before. Although she is very maternal she is not one to express her emotions openly, which made these words so special. If she says nothing else again I will treasure those words and this night.

I just phoned Mary and told her about this. She said I was very privileged to be having the experience of taking care of Mum.

The Last Waltz: Love, Death & Betrayal

Wednesday 20 September 2006

When I arrived at the hospital this morning Mum told me that she wanted to be discharged. This took the hospital staff by surprise as they were clearly not prepared for her to leave today. They said lots of things had to be organized before she could go home. They needed to arrange what they called a "family meeting" where the "caregiver", who was me, gets to discuss with the relevant hospital staff all of the issues relating to the caring of a patient at home.

So the meeting was hurriedly convened in a large comfortable office. There was a social worker, a district nurse, a physiotherapist, the charge nurse, and the ward doctor. I was very impressed by this show of unity and organization, especially after Mum's comments about no two staff members having the same information about her. They then each described the issues I would have to deal with when looking after Mum at home. I threw them a curve ball by letting them know that I was considering returning to South Africa for a month, although I said I would pass on what they told me to whichever sibling came to relieve me first. What they told me was all logical and common sense and I didn't learn anything new.

They kept going on about wanting to check the house to see what alterations could be made to make it safer for Mum to negotiate. In particular they were concerned about how Mum would get in and out of the bath. But they had all met her and all appreciated that it was going to be impossible to make any adjustments because she was being very stubborn about it. Mum had told them she had developed all the techniques she needed to negotiate the way around her own house and didn't need any of these fancy gadgets that they were offering. I had been with Mum when most of these discussions took place and I knew how exasperated the hospital staff had been at her stubbornness.

I realized that some of the equipment could become useful as Mum's health deteriorated, so I arranged for it to be delivered to the house tomorrow and stored in the basement without Mum knowing. They were happy about this. They were going to send a chair that has an electric pump to raise

The Last Waltz: Love, Death & Betrayal

it, so if necessary she could be raised into the bath. They would also send a shower attachment for the bath, a raised toilet seat to go over the existing one, a walking frame, and a commode (portable toilet). It was confirmed that Mum had agreed to have more frequent visits from the district nurse, even though she declined all other social support that was offered. I gathered together the phone numbers of all the relevant people whom I might have to contact from South Africa. I can see I may have a central role to play even when I am not here.

When I got back to Mum she wanted to know in detail what had happened. She felt a little peeved that such a meeting was going on to discuss her wellbeing without her being there. On this occasion she wasn't quite so ready to let go of the control of her health. I told her everything that was discussed at the meeting, except about the delivery tomorrow.

By mid-afternoon Mum was getting quite fidgety as she wanted to go home but the discharge papers hadn't been completed. Her bag was all packed and she was dressed and waiting on her bed for the all-clear. Previously, she was quite determined to stay in hospital, but now she was resolute in wanting out as quickly as possible. I think it was appealing to have me at home for company.

As the afternoon ticked by, we started planning her escape from the hospital. We worked out all kinds of cunning tactics to get her out the main hospital door without anyone noticing. As a last resort we were even considering the window, but, before we had to move into the implementation stage, the discharge papers came. At that moment I was sitting in her room reading the newspaper while Mum was lying on her bed listening to the radio through her earphones. I said to her that we could go now. She looked up and said, "Can we wait a few minutes, please?" I asked why, since she had been so desperate to bolt, and now the gate was open. She replied, almost in a trance, "This is such a beautiful piece of music." I could faintly hear the symphony coming from her earphones. I sat down again thinking how wonderful it was that Mum could still feel such joy in life; she could still be totally captivated by these chords that seemed to be

The Last Waltz: Love, Death & Betrayal

touching her soul. I could see a reason for her to live. If the beauty of such masterful music could make her pause while wanting to escape the hospital, surely it could hold her back from wanting to exit the world?

I waited and reflected on Mum's time in hospital. I enjoyed it because Mum had no cares and was quite comical at times. She observed small things that people wouldn't normally notice. I guess this was because her enquiring mind was suddenly focused on a small room. I enjoyed the exchange of glances when hospital workers bossed her around: "Come on, dear, sit up and drink a little water now." or "Now, dear, I think it's time we took you for a little walk to the toilet."

The attitude of the staff was particularly ironic in Mum's case, because she had been a psychiatrist in a psychiatric hospital for the largest part of her working life. Most of her patients had been elderly people.

When we got home we sat for a while in the living room, staring out at the view and soaking up the peace of being back. After a while Truffle strolled through the open door. Mum gave her a call, but she headed towards me and the hands that had been feeding her the last few days. In any other context I may have been flattered, but on this occasion I was willing her to turn and jump on Mum's lap. Mum needed all the love she could get. She showed no obvious disappointment as Truffle made her decision and jumped on to my knees. I discreetly tried to give off unwelcoming signals without Mum noticing. Truffle didn't budge.

In the evening I told Mum the news that she didn't want to hear. I told her that since her health was stable, I had decided to go back to South Africa for three or four weeks. I said that I would then come back and stay with her until the end. She didn't want to say anything, but she listened. I told her I was arranging for my siblings to have overlapping weeks here while I was away, and there would be no more than a week when she would be without a family member. During that week she could go into a rest home if she didn't want a stranger looking after her. We didn't discuss this further.

The Last Waltz: Love, Death & Betrayal

Mum is now snug in her own bed which is once again piled with books, newspapers, magazines, and her hand-scribbled notes. The TV is still on since we were watching our British dramas again. She is slowly knitting another wool hat. Things seem to be back to normal, except that she is not eating. I keep offering her the liquid drinks she enjoys, telling her that she will dehydrate if she doesn't keep drinking, but she only has small sips. She said categorically that she does not want any more solid food so that she can have some control of her death. I will keep tempting her but she seems very determined. The only solid food I saw her eat in hospital was when she tried one of the puddings that were on her dinner tray. On every other occasion the lunch and dinner trays went back untouched. I just presumed that she was getting enough nourishment from the drip and from the chicken soup I made each night. I have since learnt that a drip is nothing more than electrolytes and water. I am surprised that they don't mix in some glucose.

I can see Mum is very sad at my decision to return to South Africa.

Thursday 21 September 2006

It is becoming very difficult for Mum to walk to the toilet and I now have to escort her. Last night I left her alone to change her colostomy bag. This is something that I have had nothing to do with, so I had to follow her instructions as to what to pack into her small black zip case. I then left her to do whatever she did, in private. I wonder if I will ever have to help her do this, or indeed do the whole procedure for her. She would hate that, and would much sooner be dead. What mother could be able to endure this humiliation?

She told me that she wouldn't need to go to the toilet during the night. However, as it turned out, at 4:30am I was woken by the sound of her dragging herself to the toilet on her own. This was no ballet performance; she was clinging desperately to each wall, trying to pull her frail body along. She had already made it past my bedroom door before I came and escorted her. She probably would have made it on her

The Last Waltz: Love, Death & Betrayal

own, but it was a huge effort, and the potential for falling was high.

I am shocked at how frail Mum has become now. This is particularly noticeable when she tries to stand or walk. Her trips to the toilet symbolize her loss of independence, more than anything else, and are embarrassing for her. I have managed to turn these trips into a playful ritual. When she needs to go I ask her if I can have the pleasure of a dance. I then lift her up so that she is standing only lightly on her own legs and announce which ballroom dance it will be. We then move together, in time to a fox trot, tango or waltz. When we get to the turn in the hallway, I lead her through a spin turn. She appreciates the fact that I take the dance timing seriously, not making a mockery of the circumstances. She taught me to waltz when I was a small boy; it is time to return the favor. When we pass the grandfather clock we stop and she pulls the weight chain back to the top to keep the clock ticking.

There were several visitors today. Firstly a man came to deliver the equipment from the hospital. It was a clandestine operation and he phoned me on my cell phone when he was outside the house. We met in the street to unload the equipment, and then very quietly crept down the side of the house to put it in the basement. If Mum had looked out the window she would have been surprised to find us moving furniture around in the garden.

The next visitor was the district nurse. A nurse is now going to come three times a week to lend her assistance. Mum still doesn't want it but I am happy to have someone come so often. At least it means an objective outsider can monitor her health. The hospital's awareness of Mum's existence is one of the good things to come from her hospitalization.

My nieces came to visit next. They are quite devoted to their grandmother, but their generation seems to struggle to know what to say to older people. It is as if the art of communication by speech has now been transformed into cell phone text messages, emails, and mumbled monosyllables. It's actually funny that I sometimes find it hard to decipher their lingo. It's like tuning into a foreign language radio station. Does that mean I am now technically as well as socially separated from today's teen generation? Perhaps I've just been out of the country for too many years.

After they had left Mum said, "I can't understand them. I have lived too long."

I wonder if she realizes how profound her comment is. Mum vomited tonight. I hope this is not going to become a pattern.

Friday 22 September 2006

Soon after I woke Mum she said, "You know how concerned I have always been about the consequences of so many environmental issues? I now fear that the single biggest factor that will destroy the fabric of the society I have known is this electronic technology that has consumed the world."

I asked, "How can you make such a judgment when you are so totally detached from it?"

She replied, "That is why."

I think she is wrong, but I know where she is coming from. She ponders matters in the light of death in a way that most of us don't.

The issue most important for me right now is how to manage the toilet routine. It is becoming very stressful. This morning I told Mum about the commode in the basement and I pleaded with her to let me bring it into her room, just in case she didn't have the strength to walk. She eventually agreed as long as I covered it with a pile of her clothes, so her visitors would think it was a normal chair.

Having finally made the decision to return to Cape Town, and having informed Mum, I am now having second thoughts although I haven't told Mum about my indecision. I can't leave this much longer as my flight is next week.

Should I return to South Africa, leaving my siblings to care for Mum, and run the risk of her dying while I am gone? Or delay my decision a few more weeks, by which time it could be even harder? Or do I just commit myself to staying here with the possibility that my very presence could keep Mum going indefinitely, even though I can't stay so long?

The Last Waltz: Love, Death & Betrayal

I think I will wait and decide after I have spoken to Mary. I must say I am now very comfortable in Dunedin and the necessity of going back to Cape Town for a few weeks is less urgent. I no longer feel as if I am on holiday or visiting. I now feel as if I live here. Cape Town is becoming a memory.

Mum speaks to me every day about taking her own life. She does it very carefully and gently as she knows how sad I will be to lose her. I have accepted that she should be allowed to end her life if she is suffering but she wants to go before it gets to that. I told her that she should end her life only if there was really no enjoyment left. She told me that was now. I should have reminded her of that moment in hospital when she wanted to wait a few more minutes to listen to the music. I hope that when my sisters arrive on the weekend, she will have more reason to keep going, though one of the reasons she is keen to see Mary is to discuss, with a medical family member, how to end her life. She wants to ask what she should take and how much, even though I am certain that Mary will not pass on such information.

I explained to Mum my view that the soul moves on after death and reaches a higher level after each life, gaining more and more wisdom with each one. I have also told her that I intuitively felt that to take your own life might lead to some kind of penalty on the other side. I said that it was ironic that most religious beliefs tell you that you are going to a marvelous place after death, but the one thing that you can do to get yourself there a little quicker is the one thing that will stop you getting there at all. Such theories hold no place with Mum. I also said that in extreme circumstances I thought the penalty for suicide would not be imposed, such as those who leapt from the windows of the World Trade Centre rather than be consumed by fire, and perhaps also for elderly people suffering a painful and imminent death.

Today Mum had only four cups of fluid. All but one of these cups was water, the other being her coffee in the morning. I don't think you can live for long on a cup of coffee a day.

The Last Waltz: Love, Death & Betrayal

PART TWO

Death

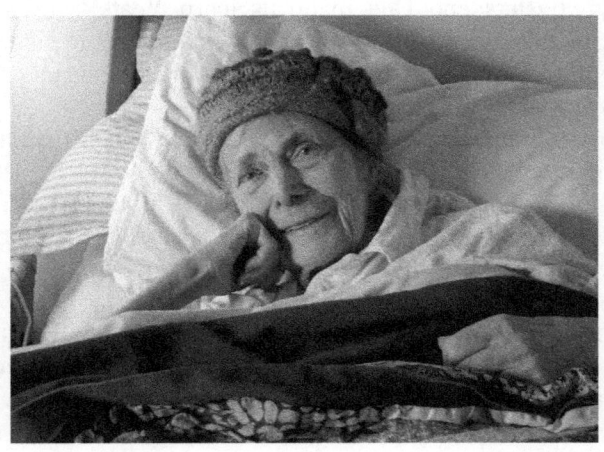

Death, death; oh, amiable, lovely death! Come, grin on me, and I will think thou smilest.

Henry VIII
Act 1V

The Last Waltz: Love, Death & Betrayal

Saturday 23 September 2006
Day one of only water: four cups.

This morning I told Mum that she was "a paltry thing, a tattered coat upon a stick."

She was quick to reply, "Unless my soul claps its hands and sings louder for every tatter in its mortal dress." This brought back memories of those painful sessions when we were youngsters and Dad made us learn Yeats' works by heart. She then added, "But my soul does not want to sing."

I replied, "And your mind does not want to consider that you have a soul."

I love Mum's constant supply of quotes. When I became more literate it was always a challenge for one of us to start a well-known quote and the other to finish it. Even as recently as my last visit here, Mum was choosing passages for me to learn by heart, and would occasionally put my learning to the test. I was still getting homework from my mother.

I am feeling so much pain as I watch Mum slowly fading away. I wonder if this will have any lasting effect on me; I don't think so as I am emotionally strong, but it is very stressful. She just lies in bed all day waiting to die. It breaks my heart. At night after she has taken her Mogadon and gone to sleep, I sit in the darkness beside her bed and watch her. The room is full of the classical music that I put on when I turn the lights out. These Tallis symphonies from the 1500s seem like dull church music to my unappreciative ear, but there's something very moving about them nonetheless. Sitting watching her, I feel I am deliberately punishing myself as I don't need to sit here. It is as if I want to suffer. Why do I do this?

During the night I come to check on her and restart the CD. She likes to have background music through until 5am when she turns on the BBC World Service.

I now believe Mum will not last another week. She has eaten no solid food for a week, and has only a few cups of liquid a day. Today she drank only water. She has no desire to keep herself alive except to say goodbye to Jo and Mary. She told me that she won't be around to see Fergus as he isn't coming until the middle of October, and added that she thought Fergus would not be able to relate to her in her present condition.

This afternoon I said to her, "You say you know the state of your health better than anyone, but I think the time has now come when I know better than you. I can see the rate of your decline. I am now certain that you will be gone in a week."

She replied, "I know my body. I won't die so soon."

I lightened things up by adding that I was concerned that she was getting a little breathless in our last few waltzes.

I don't want my Mum to suffer, so I must let her go. It is just so instinctive to try to hold on to someone you love as long as possible, but by doing that I am prolonging her suffering. Sometimes I feel she is holding on only because I am not letting her go. She is still giving me so much pleasure. Every time I am with her she gives me these beautiful, kind smiles. Today I asked her why she can smile so easily when she is suffering so much. She replied, "They are smiles for you."

Ominous clouds are gathering on the horizon as Jo and Mary are coming tonight. Mary has made such a meal of Jo's relationship with her ex-husband, Richard.

I have decided not to tell Jo and Mary my thoughts about Mum's life expectancy. They can draw their own conclusions.

Later the same night

I escorted Mum to the toilet with a delightful tango. I left and waited for her to call me to take her back. Then I heard the crash. Mum had taken a fall and had hit her head on the wooden chair in the bathroom and blood was running down her face. I cleaned her up and got her back to her bed. I told her that the point was near where she could not be left alone in the toilet. She said she was okay and that she had just lost her balance while reaching out to pull a dead leaf off a pot plant. I told her to tell that to the traffic cop!

While we waited for Jo and Mary to arrive, Mum recounted the story of the last time my sisters were together, over six years ago. She said they started the evening making

The Last Waltz: Love, Death & Betrayal

a huge effort to put the past behind them. Both were being determinedly nice to each other with lots of polite questions and chitchat about trivial things with smiles and gestures full of goodwill. Mum said that she had had high hopes that finally a truce was going to be established. However the evening imploded dramatically out of nowhere. Mary apparently laid into Jo about a whole range of childhood issues including the fact she was Dad's favorite. Jo eventually stood up and walked out. She was living in the present and it didn't matter who was Dad's favorite; nor could she remember half of what Mary was raving about. Mum thought that perhaps too much wine had been drunk. It is hard to understand how Mary, a specialized psychiatrist, should still be obsessed about what happened twenty years ago.

This incident is now at the forefront of Mum's mind as Jo and Mary have not met since that stormy evening. I think this type of family saga could be enough to keep Mum clinging on to life to learn the next enthralling episode. The drawback of living in Cape Town is that I get to hear about these dramatics only second-hand.

The Melbourne contingent, Mary with her youngest daughter, and the West Coast contingent, Jo with Orlando, arrived within two minutes of each other. I had not seen Orlando for eight years and got quite a shock to meet this tall, strong man (he was seventeen when I last saw him). Mary's daughter was in tears as she came in the door. I gave her a big hug. Jo and Mary were quite cordial towards each other.

They all walked in together to greet Mum. I went in first and announced who was entering so she didn't struggle to recognize all the faces at once. I then left them for about ten minutes to make the room less crowded.

When I returned, I could see Mum welcomed my presence. The conversation was not flowing smoothly, which often happens when you haven't seen someone for a long time. Mum also seemed to perceive Orlando as a stranger since she hadn't seen him since he went on his world travels. He has really been transformed since then. So I took my seat on the bed and tried to keep the conversation flowing. I often had to act as interpreter for Mum, because Jo and Orlando have the Kiwi tendency of speaking quickly with poor articulation. Mary has quite elegant diction. Eventually Mum was getting tired of making conversation and did her little trick of pretending to doze off. I then went closer and looked in her eyes, and she gave me that little wink to say, "Isn't this a fun way of drawing the conversation to an end?" I gave her one back, and suggested to everyone that Mum be left to snooze.

It was very late as I watched Mum dozing off. I am sure she felt it was "mission accomplished" for her. She wanted to see her daughters before she died, and although she won't wait to say goodbye to Fergus, she feels she can now die having brought closure to her life. I was happy that Jo and Mary had greeted Mum without any open hostility between them. The last thing I wanted Mum to witness in her life was her two daughters having a go at each other. I also felt I had accomplished something.

Jo is staying here at Mum's place while Mary is staying in town with one of her daughters. Since Jo is staying over for only three nights I see no need to rope her into Mum's nighttime needs. Although I would appreciate having a good night of undisturbed sleep, Mum and I have a comfortable routine.

At 4am I awoke and went to Mum's room. I thought I would wake her and see if she wanted to go to the toilet. When I got there she already had the light on and the blankets pulled back, waiting for me. How did she know I was coming? It was a very cold night and she would hardly be up and waiting if I wasn't coming. I am really watching out for mental telepathy now, after the incident in the hospital. I feel that Mum and I are really connected; we seem to think alike on everything. This is especially the case when other people are around. Maybe this just comes from living in close proximity for seven weeks and in a situation where she is becoming quite dependent on me.

I am incredibly exhausted from lack of real sleep.

The Last Waltz: Love, Death & Betrayal

Sunday 24 September 2006
Day two of only water: four cups.

Mary has a dim view of the alleged relationship between Richard and Jo a year or so ago. Because of this, Mary's children seem unsure how to react to Jo and her son. Orlando is like a Roman boy who left for battle, and after many years of conquering the world has returned as a worldly-wise warrior. He is tall, handsome and confident.

Mary came back to Broad Bay during the morning, and my sisters and I sat around chatting most of the day. It was a warm, sunny day and we were able to sit outside for a change. We took turns at popping in to chat with Mum. I was an absolute zombie from last night's duty. When I took Mum to the bathroom at lunchtime, she was totally breathless. We are going to have to cut out the spin turns in the waltz. In reality, I think our last waltz is near.

During the afternoon Mum presented us with her handwritten "Living Will." It was not a total surprise since we had heard her express its contents many times. The will stated her desire to have no further medical treatment and to be allowed to stop eating and to choose when to stop taking fluids. After we had each read it, she asked if we would respect her wishes.

We all did.

I decided I was not going to return to South Africa.

As a doctor, she must have known how easy it is to keep people alive for years and years if you put them in hospital and medicate them. Such a prospect filled her with horror, with images of the psychiatric patients she had treated for so many years. Mum's big fear is Mary taking control of her life when she no longer has the mental faculties to express her desires. Last year she changed her medical power of attorney from Mary to me for this reason.

LIVING WILL
Sept 2006

To whom it may concern:
And to my children: Fergus Davison, Mary Davison, Jo Ewer, Sean Davison.

I am ill with progressive cancer that can only get worse. My quality of life can only deteriorate. I do not wish to have a protracted disagreeable death, and I think I can count on all of you in supporting me in this. I have decided to die by inanition (unless alternative means occur), and would like to make the following request:

No resuscitation (or ECT).
No antibiotics.
No attempts to make me eat.
I wish to be the one to decide when I stop fluids.
I would prefer as few people to know about this as possible.
(It is what I call a "Bobby Sands.")
I would like to thank everyone for their help up till now. Sean, what would I have done without you!
P.E. Davison

The Last Waltz: Love, Death & Betrayal

> LIVING WILL   Sept 2006
> To whom it may concern:
> And to: My children:
> Fergus Davison, Philippa Davison
> Joanna Ewer, Sean Davison:
> I am ill with a progressive
> cancer which can only get worse
> My quality of life can only
> deteriorate, I do not
> wish for a protracted
> disagreeable Death, and
> I think I can count on
> all of you in supporting
> me in this. I have decided
> to die by inanition
> (unless attenative means
> occur) And would like to
> make the following
> Requests:
>
> No resuscitation (or eject)
> No antibiotics
> No attempts to make me eat
> I wish to be the one to
> decide when I stop fluids
>
> I would prefer as few
> people to know about this
> as possible
>
> (It is what I call a Bobby
> Sands)
>
> I would like to thank every-
> one for their help up till now
> Sean, what would I have
> done without you!
>   P.E. Davison

The Last Waltz: Love, Death & Betrayal

I went for a long walk and thought about Mum's Will. I had to look up in the dictionary what "inanition" meant. She had very deliberately and carefully planned every word. She had probably been working on it for days, which in itself surprised me, since I have been watching over her for so much of the time. Also, her ability to write is very limited with her wobbly right hand. She had even written a rough draft in pencil, which was almost identical. It must have been a huge mental and physical effort of concentration and stamina for her. This was driven by her overwhelming determination to end her life. I was really taken aback to discover what had been going on without my knowledge. To my face she was going through the daily motions of being interested in life, but behind this facade she had been determinedly composing this Living Will to emphatically state the desire that was constantly on her mind.

She didn't want there to be any doubts. There was no arguing her resolve now.

This legal document stated that should she lose her mental faculties, her power of attorney went to me. This included the authority to decide whether a life support system could be turned off. This document was drawn up shortly after she returned from visiting Mary in Melbourne, where she found Mary unsympathetic to the pain she had. She told me she tried not to tell Mary if she was in pain because Mary was so brash and unsympathetic, even though it was Mary's medical opinion she most wanted. When this medical power of attorney was drawn up, she said openly that I had a kinder heart than Mary and she would be happier to know that if she did lose her mental faculties, I would use my heart to make the best decision about her future. She said there was no telling what Mary might do. At that time she even added that Mary might pull the plug too soon on her, although right now I think that would be a wonderful outcome in Mum's eyes.

In the evening I chatted to Mum about her will. I told her we agreed that it was her decision and that her course of action seemed reasonable. She probably wouldn't have long to go, and that we would not send her away, or force medication or food on her. I then questioned a small detail. I suggested she delete the line, "unless alternative means occur." She said no alternative means would occur if her Living Will is honored and she is left to die her "Bobby Sands" way, a hunger strike. I agreed with her and admired how carefully she had planned her death. Since God wasn't going to help her to a quick and pain-free death, she would take the matter into her own hands. Her plan really is foolproof and her resolve will win her this last battle in life.

I asked her if she felt shame in going on a hunger strike and for this reason wanted as few people to know as possible. She quickly replied, "Not at all, I am only worried that, if too many people find out, there will be someone who will try to stop me." This made sense to me because she had been telling many people her plan to stop eating for some weeks now.

I then asked her how she felt about other elderly women with cancer who choose to live as long as they can.

She said that that was their choice.

I suggested to her that they could be offended by her implication that life is not worth living when they get to a comparable stage.

She replied, "The time comes when life is not worth living. They will come to the same conclusion as me one day." Then she added, "I prefer life to death. But this is not life."

Finally there is absolutely no question now that I am going to stay with Mum to the end. I don't need to seek advice from anyone. I can see how quickly she is fading. Even though I told Mum that I am definitely not leaving, she didn't seem to believe me. This is not surprising since she has watched my indecision for so long (I wonder if she calls me "Either/Or" The Second.) I repeated it to her several times during the day so she had no doubts.

Today she got her Living Will initiative off to an emphatic start as not only did she not take in any solid foods, but the liquids amounted to only four glasses of water. I did offer her some potato soup heated up from last week. She asked if it had been cooked with meat. I said no, as I wanted her to have the extra nutrients. She said, "But it must have meat in it because you cooked it with a chop last week, you told me." She didn't forget; I guess her world is so small now that she will notice these little things.

I remember Mum once described how the size of people's worlds determined how obsessive they were. She said people who live in small worlds are so focused on the little things around them that these insignificant details become very big, and when the people who have big worlds enter them they will easily cause offence if they underestimate the importance of the things in the lives of the "small-world" people.

The important message tonight is that I must remember that Mum's shrunken world will catch me out if I try to trick her into taking nourishment that she doesn't want. She has all day to think about so few things and will catch me out every time. She also has time to think of ways to be mischievous.

Monday 25 September 2006
Day three of only water: four cups.

Things are starting to unravel at every turn. Last night with Mum was scary. As with the previous night, I randomly got up to check on her on several occasions. The first couple of times she was sound asleep and I just restarted her CD. On the third occasion around 5am I found her straddled between her bed and the commode, one arm propping herself up on the bed, the other holding on to the commode, unable to move. Her next action would have been to fall to the floor between the bed and commode. I rescued her in time, and told her that she must call out for me if she wants me to come and help. I also gave her an old cowbell that she had when she was a girl, telling her to ring it any time she needed me since I couldn't always hear her calling.

I was woken again later in the morning after a dreadful night's sleep by Fergus's phone call. He calls every Monday morning. Mum revealed her Living Will request to him; he agreed to it. When I spoke to him after he had finished speaking to Mum, he said that he agreed with it only to please Mum, but thought it totally unnecessary. He asked if I thought she would live a reasonable life if she started eating again. I said that I thought she would, and would probably get back to the state she was in when I arrived. Fergus said she should eat and that it was appalling what Mum planned to do. I agreed with him from his perspective, but if he were here with Mum he would understand why she was doing it. Fergus forthrightly repeated that she was crazy to do this. Perhaps he is right.

I am feeling reassured, knowing that Mum will never be alone again now that I am staying here. The end of her life will be a happy time, surrounded by family. I could not bear for Mum to end her life as lonely as she was before I came back. I still recall those daily phone calls when I was in Cape Town. I could feel the loneliness and misery in her heart. I now can't believe it took me so long to cancel my plans to return to Cape Town. I caused Mum such fear and uncertainty at the prospect of my going back. She must have really fretted. Would she have to go into a rest home? Would she die alone? It must have been horrible for her. Although she never expressed these concerns openly to me, I heard just enough snippets of her conversations with the nurses to know what emotional turmoil she was going through. I admonish myself for letting her suffer like that.

Mum is the type of person who would have loved to have been surrounded by close family all her life. But I think the quote goes, "Children don't belong to us, they belong to life." That was certainly the case with our family. I guess the main reason things didn't work out the way she wanted is that her family-orientated genes were diluted by Dad's gypsy ones. Dad's quote was always, "A tree that grows alone grows strongest." Those words illustrate our family in that we have all dispersed to different corners of the world. Of course our parents are partly to blame for our dispersal. They immigrated to such a remote corner of the planet where we were almost certainly going to want to spread our wings and find the larger world. I know I have a good dose of Dad's independence genes. I need a lot of time on my own to maintain my inner peace and harmony. Fergus is the same; he has been living alone for the last thirty years. Neither of us has married nor lived for any significant length of time with a partner. Jo and Mary are different. Although Jo has chosen a rather reclusive lifestyle living in a house above the beach, on the remote West Coast, I think she is quite dependent on human company, as Mum is. Without any doubt, Mary thrives on being surrounded by people.

Perhaps this difference is a male/female thing. I think men in general need a lot more space than women. After all, we did evolve from cave dwellers where the male spent much of his time roaming the prairies, hunting for wild game to bring home to his woman who was nursing the baby cave dwellers. Not much has changed since then, apart from women now sharing the hunting role.

So should I feel guilty for not having spent more of my adult life with my mum? I feel guilty right now, but in reality children should be free to move on, to discover life and discover themselves, and mothers should accept that. I moved on. It is also part of the pioneering spirit that is so strong in humankind. This resulted in humans leaving Africa and colonizing the world, and more recently space. If we try to suppress this instinct we are suppressing the very instinct that has made humankind what it is today. When I discussed this with Mum, she felt that we have progressed too far. She thinks we should in fact go back a hundred years to where we had horses and carts and bicycles; before we had telephones, where human values really were treasured. I feel that the direction humankind is taking is determined by natural selection of our genes. Whatever dreadful life awaits us will be a consequence of the same genetic processes that got us where we are today; this cannot be stopped.

I think fathers are possibly satisfied when their children grow up and move out of the nest. This would fit in with my theory about males wanting more space. I wonder how I will feel in old age. Will I want to have space or be surrounded by family?

So many people are quick with the line that you must get married and have children "because you don't want to be alone in old age." I wonder if this is really the case, or are we just projecting ourselves into the future when we look at old people and think how horrible it would be to be alone at that stage of life? Perhaps many old people enjoy being alone. I will find out some day.

The Last Waltz: Love, Death & Betrayal

Mum has stopped getting up now. She didn't get up yesterday or today. She just doesn't have the strength to waste energy on getting dressed and moving around the house, even for the pleasure of going back to bed later. Everything is a huge effort for her. I was very scared at how breathless she was when I took her to the toilet this afternoon. We were doing only a very slow fox trot.

For dinner I decided I wanted to eat on my own, away from the family at home. I am exhausted and stressed; I just need time alone. I drove into town and went to my favorite Chinese restaurant near the hospital. This place is always crowded with students and you are expected to share a table. This never worries me as I always feel completely anonymous.

After I had placed my order at the counter I went and sat down to relax and feel free of family stresses. The woman next to me tapped me on the shoulder and said, "Hello, Uncle Sean!" It was my eldest niece with a male friend. "What are you going to have for dinner, Sean?" I told her I had to change my order quickly to have extra chilies. I dashed up to the counter and told the lady to make mine a takeaway.

This evening Mum asked me how Mary and Jo are getting along. I told her they both seem to be making a big effort and that harmony is prevailing. She said she still feels responsible for her daughters' latest fallout over Richard's relationship with Jo. Even though it had been several years since he divorced Mary, it did put Mum in a very uncomfortable position.

But what else could she have done? Richard so gallantly came to her and requested permission to date her younger daughter. Such courtesy seems a little comical these days, but I have to admire Richard's gentlemanly behavior. How could Mum have refused? They were both middle-aged and seemed to know what they were doing.

Mary was very upset when she heard about this and didn't speak to Mum for a couple of weeks. I remember Mum was in a state of agitation over her silence. I emailed Mary and pleaded with her to start phoning Mum again.

The Last Waltz: Love, Death & Betrayal

Anyway, Mum is happier to know that it seems to have blown over and her condoning of this relationship is history. I just hope it stays peaceful for a few more days until Jo goes.

Later the same night

God almighty, I can't believe what happened tonight. What the hell is Mary playing at, she must be insane!

Sarah just rocked up at the door unannounced, apparently invited by Mary! I haven't seen her for about 25 years. I don't know what has happened to her in the last twenty-five years.

I only know that she still lives in Dunedin. Sarah's a lesbian, but that's hardly the point. The point is that she's the lesbian partner that Mary "stole" from Jo when Sarah and Jo were in a stable relationship decades ago. Mary had a fling with her because she wanted to hurt Jo, not because she had any genuine lesbian tendencies.

Today Mary probably just wanted to put the boxing gloves on. But Jo is non-confrontational so she ignored the provocation and instead consumed another bottle of wine. There's no doubt that Mary invited her to today as revenge for Jo's relationship with Richard.

And that wasn't even the end of it.

Along came the crooked hand of fate and Richard turned up! He came with my two nieces because they happened to be passing by. My God, it couldn't have been scripted better.

The wine flowed. The air was thick. The nieces were tense. Mary was wound up. Jo was pissed off. Richard was a meek mouse... and oh, by the way... Mum was lying in her death bed in the next room.

I think there can be little doubt that our family will dissolve after Mum's death.

Tuesday 26 September 2006
Day four of only water: four cups.

I am slipping into a horrible depression. I am really grieving at the coming loss of Mum. I know it is not logical, and that I must accept that a woman of eighty-five has lived to a good age and will die soon. I should be celebrating her life and not mourning her loss.

It is not healthy to sit in her room at night, with that bleak music penetrating my heart, encouraging the tears to flow. I don't know what has come over me. But it is getting worse. I came home from my swim and sat with Mum on her bed. I just had to tell her how much pain I was feeling. She had been the loving mother I had turned to all my life, with any pain or hurt I had. Now she is the cause of my pain and I cannot turn to her. I had been avoiding turning to her for sympathy. I had kept showing her my strength, to make her passage to death easier, trying to show her I was willing to let nature take its course and let her go.

I sat down and didn't hold back. I told her openly that I was suffering terribly at the prospect of her dying soon. I tried to control my tears. She reached out and held me to comfort me as if I was still her blue-eyed boy, telling me it was all right. Of course it wasn't all right. How could it be when these mother's arms would soon be cold with death, the calming words silenced forever, the smiling face a memory, and the future empty of her seemingly immortal presence? I cried it all out. She just kept comforting me. Something like this had not happened since I was a boy. It felt so reassuring. It also felt strange that she should be comforting me when she was the one who really was in need of support. Mum was heading into the totally unknown experience of death, unaware of how it would happen or whether she would suffer, and what was on the other side.

I tried changing tack and told her that I would be strong for her. I said it was my duty to keep a "stiff upper lip." I told her I would try to focus on celebrating her life. Poor Mum, she couldn't say anything that would ease my pain. Her future is cast in stone, mine is far from certain. I tried to pull myself together for her sake. I was being selfish, seeking her sympathy at a time like this.

Mum said it must be horrible for me to watch her fading away. I said it was actually easier to share her journey to death than be phoned in Cape Town to be told that she had died. Mum's slow suffering death has saved me this pain. I

The Last Waltz: Love, Death & Betrayal

am sure she didn't see it that way. A sudden heart attack would have been a blessing. It is such a twisted fate.

When I left her room I felt some relief. I had let my emotions out, and I think it did Mum no harm to know how I was suffering. It gives her further proof of how loved she is, as if she ever doubted it.

I know that it will only be after she dies that I will truly discover the value of her love.

I have now come to my room to calm down and write my journal. To write is better than to cry. Jo and Mary were aware of what was happening in Mum's room. They know how close I am to her and I suppose they realize that I have been living Mum's life for so long now that I am bound to have such an emotional bond with her.

Later the same day

I am exhausted from lack of sleep, and that is why I am losing control of my emotions. Really I must get some solid sleep. The only solution seems to be to become a Mogadon junky as these pills still work well. I swim most days but this is not enough to knock me out. Once my subconscious comes to the fore in the night I can't stop reliving every minute I spent with Mum the previous day.

Jo and Orlando leave tomorrow. I know they would like to spend more time with me since we have seen so little of each other in recent years, but I am not in a good frame of mind to be chatting about our own lives which seem so trivial when Mum lies dying in the next room. I know I can't blame Jo. There is no reason she has to be in the same state of mind as I am. We both have different feelings towards Mum, as we did towards Dad. I know Jo felt a lot more pain when Dad died.

Jo and I talked about him yesterday. We both missed him when he died because he had had such a huge impact in our lives. He was an incredible disciplinarian, but he also had a wonderful sense of humor. He brought us up like soldiers, under total control of his piercing bright blue eyes and booming, deep voice. One of Jo's favorite memories of him was his Sunday morning drill of "Captain's rounds" when he would inspect the cleanliness of our bedrooms. He would put a stick under his arm, white glove on his hand, and stroll around the room wiping his gloved finger across every hidden surface looking for dust. He had been an officer in the British Army so this discipline came very easily to him. This performance could be seen as absurd, but was only the tip of an iceberg of total control.

I reminisced about my most lasting memory of Dad. It was the very formal evening dinners. Dad would ring a bell ten minutes before dinner so we could smarten our clothes and wash our hands. The men (and boys) of the house would then stand by their chairs at the dinner table until all the women were seated. We would have a very structured meal using the finest family crockery and silver, with four candles in silver candlestick-holders burning in the center of the table. Dad would direct the discussion from the head of the table. If there was a knock at the door or the phone rang during the meal, we were to ignore it. He said we had to assume at all times that we were eating at the officers' dining table. Throughout the meal there was a strict code of conduct about how we held our knives and forks, how often we put them down during the meal, how the food had to be kept within a certain distance from the side of the plate, the angle at which we left our knives and forks when we were still eating or when we had finished, and, most importantly, we all had to finish eating at about the same time. And this was only dinner table conduct.

Why Jo felt so much closer to Dad than Mum is a mystery to me when Mum supplied the love and affection that we didn't receive from him. It could have been because she was his favorite. Now, at Mum's deathbed, she feels only token loss. It is just hard for me having her here when I know she doesn't feel the same pain as I do.

Although it bugs me that she and Orlando are just hanging around at a loose end, I shouldn't be so hard on her since I have not given her a job to help me with. I am totally absorbed in the task of nursing Mum, and need no help, and expect no help. At the same time I also have to acknowledge that Mum is Jo's mother too and she has as much right as me to be here, and certainly needs to be here to say goodbye. I also have to be sensitive to the fact that Mum wants to say goodbye to all her children, although she does confide that it is very difficult to find things to talk about with Jo.

In the afternoon I spoke to Mum about getting some morphine. Mum didn't think it possible to get much. She repeated that her best strategy was to take her destiny into her own hands by not eating and just fading away quickly. She is lost for an explanation as to why it is taking so long.

Mum started her water-only diet on Saturday. I think that once since she saw Jo and Mary, she felt that was her cue to stop eating. I carefully keep an eye on the amount she drinks as I don't want her to start vomiting again. She is certainly weakening each day. I joke with her that I am keeping accurate records of her fluid intake because I want to write a scientific paper on her death. She has a lot of respect for me as a scientist and takes it seriously, allowing me to measure carefully the volume of each cup of water I give her.

For the first time last night she realized that she was too weak to use the normal toilet. She has actually been too weak for several days now, as I was almost carrying her on these walks, with her feet barely resting on the ground, pretending that she was still dancing with me. We had to stop periodically for her to catch her breath. She has now accepted that she must use the commode next to her bed every time. She calls me when she wants to go and I carefully lift her on to it, trying to protect her modesty throughout the procedure. I stoically empty the commode as soon as she has finished.

I keep probing Mum on her thoughts about the future. It is very clear-cut as she wants only one thing: to die. But I want to know if she is curious about the things that have captured her mind for so many years, things that are still unfolding in the news each day. How does she feel about not knowing what will become of the anarchy in Iraq? Who will become the next president of the USA? What will become of global warming, overpopulation, the end of oil, and the dumbing down of society? She said she no longer cares, certainly not enough to keep living. She added that most of these issues will carry on forever and I will one day be in the same position as she is now, where I will have to switch off and let them continue without me. I asked her if she was sad not

The Last Waltz: Love, Death & Betrayal

knowing what will become of her children and grandchildren, not to find out if I will have children, if Jo will find happiness, or if Fergus will move to New Zealand. Will Mary marry Nigel? Will the family base move to Melbourne? Mum said, "I am letting go to a new family order now and Fergus will be the head."

But she does seem to enjoy each day, each visitor, and each different event. Her greatest sadness now is the loss of reading ability. This has been more of a blow than when she stopped being able to paint.

Jo is leaving tomorrow, so tonight we took the last opportunity to go for a walk together. She was feeling sentimental and said that after I return to Cape Town it was possible we might never see each other again, and she didn't think I would come back to New Zealand. The thought of not seeing Jo again hadn't crossed my mind but I guess it is a possibility.

I told Jo I was sure we would meet many more times. We have always been the closest siblings because we grew up together, and the bond we had would always be there. I told her how she had shaped my life so much as a teenager. Even though she was a year older and much more mature than me, she felt no embarrassment taking me wherever she and her friends went. Jo was cool and very good looking; I was neither. I felt honored to hang out with her. I learnt so much about life and myself that would have taken many years to learn on my own. She really didn't appreciate the impact she had had on my early life. She agreed we had a close bond and said she could see it in letters she still has from me. She commented on the fact that we had once been on totally different ends of the political spectrum, when I was a National Party candidate and she was a free-living hippy in the bush. Yet it made absolutely no difference to our friendship. She knew I would see the light one day.

Although Jo drinks a lot she still manages to run ten kilometers most mornings. I was struggling to keep up walking with her tonight. At one point she wanted to pee, so she lifted her skirt and did so in someone's front garden (it was getting dark). Although Jo now has a respectable job as a teacher and has come out of the bush, it seems the bush has

The Last Waltz: Love, Death & Betrayal

not come out of her. She could never offend me as she does everything so naturally, and she never seems to be angry with anyone. Although we are quite different people now, we will always be very close.

I mentioned to Jo that the family speculates that she may be a budding alcoholic, since she downs a lot of wine every time we see her. She refuted this suggestion emphatically. She said she always drinks a lot when family is around because it is a special occasion. I have my doubts. It's in the genes, but at least alcohol makes her relaxed and cheerful.

Jo thought Dad's alcoholism wasn't always a bad thing, as a lot of fun was created along the way. She reminded me of how, on St Patrick's Day every year, Dad used to invite the priests from the Hokitika monastery around for a few drinks after dinner. By breakfast time he would take them home totally inebriated. I wondered why he partied with Catholic priests when he was a diehard Protestant from Northern Ireland. Jo thought it was simply because he was always looking for an excuse to party. I suspect he more enjoyed getting one over the Catholic Church. I thought the family parties were a good thing; they were always highly entertaining. Dad would recharge our glasses all night. I used to keep disposing of my wine into the vases Mum had strategically left around the living room. After one party when I got up during the night to go to the toilet, I popped into the kitchen to empty the vase. As it happened Dad heard me, followed me into the kitchen and caught me in the act. I was standing naked at the kitchen sink, a bouquet of flowers in one hand and a vase in the other, pouring red wine down the sink. I am sure he thought I was a chip off the old block. On another occasion when Richard stayed over on his own, he heard Richard get up and go outside and urinate in the garden. Dad got up and locked the door and windows and went back to bed, leaving Richard to sleep outside.

It must have been public knowledge that Dad was a bit of a drinker, especially after he made it on to the front page of the *Truth* newspaper. The banner headline read: "Doc Pours Doc's Blood Down Sink." This article described how a Hokitika doctor had "accidentally" poured the blood, drawn from Dad after he had been stopped for drinking and driving, down the sink. Fortunately Dad was honorable enough to admit guilt without the blood test, to prevent his colleague from facing charges. This incident was a big blow to his pride and drove him to the bottle some more.

Jo also told me that she didn't have an intimate relationship with Richard. She said he had pursued her but she only wanted friendship. We agreed it was no one else's business anyway, especially not Mary's, since they divorced many years ago. Mary just blew the whole incident out of proportion.

Perhaps Jo is right and I will not return. But I do know I will stay in touch with her regardless. I am now thinking of so many more things I should have asked her on our walk tonight. I would like to know more about her fragile relationship with Mary. Richard's little cameo performance did nothing to mend their sisterly love, which must already have been beyond repair. I suppose there will be time to talk to her tomorrow.

Fergus and I are just so damned boring. It's hard to believe we are related to our sisters. Perhaps we need to get out a bit more.

Wednesday 27 September 2006
Five days of only water: four cups.

I had a troubled sleep last night, after so much reminiscing about Dad. I didn't get the chance to say goodbye to him, and I regret it to this day. Although I didn't have much love for him he had a huge impact on my upbringing. In many ways his ending had parallels with Mum's. He was at death's door and I had the chance to fly over in time to say my goodbyes.

I chose not to. I knew what I was doing, but I didn't know how I would feel later.

The district nurse spoke to me in the garden today. She told me that Mum wants me to tell her she can die, and that I have to be strong and let Mum decide when to go. She said that this is a common trend seen in dying people: they often hold on, even if they are suffering, because they are trying to delay the hurt that their death will cause.

The Last Waltz: Love, Death & Betrayal

Jo and Orlando left today, sporting big hangovers. Before Jo left she told me that Mum had asked her to leave today, even though she was willing to stay longer. I told Jo that I thought Mum really wanted Orlando to leave, and not her. Mum had told me she felt Orlando was a strange man in the house and she wanted to be surrounded by familiarity. It is better that Orlando doesn't find this out. He was a very charming boy: innocent, funny, and very beautiful. He is now a sweet man in a strong, muscular body. Mum is just not in a state of mind where she can rediscover the boy she knew and loved from eight years ago; whereas, Orlando's devotion towards her never changed, even while his body underwent this metamorphosis.

My youngest niece has returned to Melbourne to go back to school. She was really cut up seeing her grandmother dying.

Mary has blown in. It would have been possible to squeeze Jo and Mary into the house at the same time, but they were both quite aware that this could have led to a boil over. I now wonder how we will get on.

We can't really be sure how long Mum has left, and Mary and I will both stay until her death. Mum said to me that Mary wanted to be here for her last breath, and felt obliged to give her that wish. We will just have to anticipate when it is coming so we can make sure we are both with her at the time. We are going to make sure one of us is at home all the time.

I am a little nervous about Mary being so domineering and decisive that she might push Mum in the death direction when she may not be quite ready. She has commented several times that Mum should be hurried along. Mary doesn't mean this in a horrible way, as she will feel Mum's loss as much as me; she just thinks it will be in everyone's best interest to end this protracted death bed scene.

This afternoon I picked up Mum's first morphine prescription. She can get only a week's supply at a time. When Mary found out I had it, I could see she was annoyed I hadn't told her immediately.

Mum had a really perky day today with three visitors. The most entertaining was John Francis who particularly enjoys visiting when Jo and Mary are here, since they are both crazy about his art. He phoned yesterday to say he had enough petrol to come today. To his credit, he has always been exceptionally reliable in sticking to his visiting plans. He did a sketch of Mum while he sat with her. I couldn't see much resemblance to her, or even to a human being, for that matter. We all told him how amazing the sketch was.

In the evening Mum acknowledged that each day gives her some pleasure, but continues to profess that she wants to die sooner rather than later. I casually mentioned that I had a week's supply of morphine. She seemed uninterested. This suggested to me that she is quite happy with her daily life at present.

Thursday 28 September 2006
Day six of only water: three cups.

Today for the first time I was unable to get Mum to stand by herself. This is her sixth day of only water, and thirteenth day without solid food. It is impossible to gauge how long she has left. How long can an eighty-five-year-old live on three glasses of water a day? In spite of her frailty, it was a good day for her (I wish I could say the same about me. I suspect I am more tired than she is.) At one point in the afternoon I asked if she was happy and she said she was. This makes me feel better and encourages me to keep providing interesting things to make each day different and special. It is amazing how her brain and personality have remained unchanged even though her body is fading away.

She is on a very serene and comfortable plane now. Her most common tease is about my color-blindness. She is making quite a meal of the fact that I struggle to see red and green; throughout my life it has hardly been mentioned. She may ask me to tune her radio to the frequency marked with a red felt pen, but then she will add, "Sorry, but of course you won't be able to see the red." On another day she may ask me to get her green socks, red pills or green jersey, and each time it is followed by her well-worn joke. But she does make it sound so funny. Her mind focuses on these little things around her.

The Last Waltz: Love, Death & Betrayal

I keep telling her how contented she looks and what a nice way to end her life, with all her children staying in close contact with her, living in this charming rustic house with its beautiful, peaceful view. She agrees with me that she is very content. I tell her that if she started eating again, she could probably live another six months. She gives her standard reply that there is no point because she is going to die anyway. She says she feels bloated and would not enjoy eating again because the food tastes so unpleasant, and she always has a dull headache.

Mum often checks the time on her watch, which I find intriguing for someone who should have no concern about the time. Surely every hour is the same, especially if you are not waiting for the next meal. She often comments on how slowly time is passing, after she has checked her watch. Today she said, "It is only two pm but I was sure it would be about five." She wishes time would speed up so she could die sooner. I pointed out to her that the logic didn't quite add up. She wants to get it over with quickly, as if she has something important to do after it is done, like students who want to get the end-of-year exams over with so they can relax on holiday.

We often have discussions about other people who have survived without food for long periods of time. The main one is Bobby Sands of the Irish Republican Army, whom she is using as her reference point. We disagree on the details of his life and hunger strike. I told her that my information was correct because I was twenty at the time and was drawn into Dad's obsession with this hunger strike. He was caught in an interesting paradox. It seemed quite absurd that Dad, as an Ulster man from Northern Ireland, who had been fighting the IRA after he returned from fighting in the Second World War, should be sympathetic to this terrorist. But Bobby Sands hated the English, and Dad had also grown up with this same bitterness flowing in his blood. So from his distant view he respected Bobby Sands and hoped he would bring some damage to the British government.

Mum asked me to look up on the Internet to see how many days he survived. I did this and told her he lived for sixty-five. I added that he was a fit young man of twenty-

The Last Waltz: Love, Death & Betrayal

seven and she was a frail old lady of eighty-five, with cancer, and couldn't expect to live for more than a fraction of that time. I assured her the end was near. She told me she wasn't convinced as she felt so healthy and also couldn't understand why she never felt hungry.

We then discussed other people surviving on nothing and how long they lived, the Jews in the Nazi concentration camps, people shipwrecked on desert islands, and people drifting on the sea in lifeboats. When it became clear that people could survive for quite a long time on almost nothing, she ended the discussion with, "I don't want to talk about it."

"But Mum," I replied, and she would interrupt again with the same assertion. This became a standard conversation pattern and a joke. But it is also a very sensitive point for her. She has embarked on this hunger strike and the last thing she wants to hear is that it could last for longer than she expected. She thinks she is probably doing better than shipwrecked survivors in a life raft.

I don't think she has got more than a week to go. How many times have I thought that now? I have told Fergus this. I don't want to be responsible for his not seeing Mum alive because he didn't know how long she had left. I told him if he doesn't come immediately he will probably only be coming for her funeral. Mum would like to stay alive to say goodbye to Fergus, but if it means just hanging on in her present misery, her preference is to exit this world without Fergus's farewell. Fergus and Mum are both content in this likely outcome so there should be no regrets.

I think Fergus would prefer to be here for the funeral rather than a miserable death. He is a man who is ruled by his head and duty. It is more important for him to do what's right than what he actually wants to do. To be present at the funeral, in his opinion, is the right thing to do; as the eldest child, he will be the unofficial head of the family when Mum dies. I see Fergus as a bit like Prince Charles. Both men are very proper, have high ideals, lots of good ideas, but limited drive and leadership skills because of their very diplomatic and agreeable manner.

Richard and my nieces came for dinner tonight. During the evening, Mary was bullying Mum to take food. When I reprimanded Mary, Richard took her side and said Mum should be encouraged to eat. I was annoyed by this and reminded them that we had agreed to her Living Will. This didn't stop Mary. Later Mum told me she had pretended to drink soup to get Mary to back off. Things are getting tense between Mary and me now.

But seeing Mum at such peace is making it easier for me to let her go. It no longer seems like a clumsy stumbling towards the end. It did look like it was heading that way as she was slowly losing her independence and fighting it every step of the way, continuously trying to do things on her own that she wasn't capable of. Each step of the decline was a distressing blow for both of us. These shocks were making this journey a painful and agonizing one to withstand. But now that she has accepted her loss of independence with a charming smile and clever one-liners, we are in a surreal zone of peace and harmony. I want to savor the words of her last days. I also want to stay in the house and be near her in case she needs help. She must never feel alone now. I also feel a need to protect her from visitors who stay too long.

This is a graceful way for Mum to go. This is what she deserves. It is as if this last act has been carefully stage managed and scripted by Mum herself, as if her death is her final work of art.

Friday 29 September 2006
Day seven of only water: four cups.

Last night when I was lifting Mum from the bed on to the commode she started singing me the teapot song that she saw Ian and me singing in the wedding video: "I'm a little teapot short and stout." She then paused.

I instinctively came in with another line: "Tip me over and pour me out!"

We looked at each other and started laughing as we saw the irony of these words. It was slightly embarrassing as the words, when applied to our situation, did make her seem a little silly.

Today I had a visit from my old friend, Nina. She wanted to catch up with me and thought it appropriate to visit me at

Mum's so that I wouldn't have to leave her. When Nina arrived she greeted Mum in her room, and then sat on the balcony drinking coffee with me; occasionally Mary joined us. Nina was there for a good two hours since it was a sunny afternoon and we were catching up on all the news.

Later in the afternoon, when I went in to see Mum, she became quite demanding, asking, "When will that woman go? What is she doing here?" I found this a bit odd when Mum has so many visitors to see her. Was it that she was jealous of a woman coming to see me, and keeping me from her for so long? This suspicion was confirmed by Dr. MacDonald, who had come to see Mum while Nina was still here. He told me later that Mum was quite adamant in her complaints about Nina being in her house. Oh dear, I had better be careful not to cause further offence. That is not something I want to do.

Saturday 30 September 2006
Day eight of only water: three and a half cups.

Last night was not good. Mary can be a very cutting and insensitive person. Our crisis probably started smoldering when I showed resistance to being bossed around. I was also feeling sad at having lost the idyllic life I had before Mary came with her constant demands. The final straw was when I was going to bed and she said Nigel would be phoning after midnight from Melbourne. This meant I would be woken up, since the phone cord doesn't reach her room, but stops outside mine. I said it was not fair for me to be woken at that time, when I was struggling to sleep because of all the interruptions with Mum. She told me to "go take a Mogadon." I said I wasn't going to as I didn't want to take them unnecessarily. She asked if I wanted her to move out. I said under these circumstances of late night telephone calls I did, and suggested she stay with one of her daughters in the city. She said she would go back to Melbourne instead. I said that was also fine. She told me to tell that to Mum and see what she said. Of course I didn't want to do that, so that's where we left it.

The Last Waltz: Love, Death & Betrayal

I stayed up chatting to Mum, waiting for Nigel to phone rather than be woken later when I was asleep. Mary overheard Mum say several times to me, "Has that man phoned yet?" Mum knew what was going on and wanted me to get some sleep. She also made it clear that she was on my side. This was a bit out of character as she would normally have stayed neutral in such trivial disputes. However, I did appreciate the way she was protective and was genuinely concerned that I got enough sleep. Mum was playing the role of my guardian. I guess this was instinctive for her, as she was defending the person who is her loving protector right now. Perhaps this was unfair on Mary, but it was understandable.

When Mary surfaced this morning she said she was not happy in the house because she had arrived too soon. She said there was nothing she could do here and she felt like a fifth wheel. She didn't like the way I idolized Mum, and she didn't like the things Mum said to her. She said Mum spoke to her differently from how she spoke to me, and she was often judgmental towards her. I drove into town and bought a portable phone that Mary can keep by her bed at night. If only Mum had had one of these to prevent all those years of protracted struggles with tangled phone cables.

Mum is at quite a contented stage now, where she has stopped fighting her loss of independence and is enjoying being spoilt each day. This is a time that should be enjoyed for as long as possible, so she can die with a feeling of being loved. This is such a contrast from the crises of the last weeks.

The nurse came today. They all know about Mum's starvation plan as Mum openly discusses it with them, as if pleading with them to help her die. I had previously discussed with the nurse about when Mum should start taking her prescribed morphine. I had been told that this should happen when she was in pain. The nurse reiterated that I must let Mum know that I am willing to let her go.

I am feeling the type of desolation one feels after a relationship ends where you have lost that partner forever and constantly miss that person. Everything in Dunedin reminds me of Mum. This is especially the case when shopping, which was always such a shared experience. Now I find shopping so hard because I know Mum will never eat again. The best I can come up with is a different brand of bottled water for her to try. Even this brings no pleasure as Mum has always been insistent on drinking tap water, even in the poorest of undeveloped countries we travelled through. She said it was so her stomach could quickly acclimatize to the local bugs.

I know I am not the first to feel this way about losing a mother. Parents are the rocks of our lives. They are the ones who have always been there for us and always loved us, no matter what we did or who we were. You can never absolutely say that of anyone else in life. The next closest you will ever come to unconditional love is from your dog, even if you come home smelling of another dog. Living in a different country did not take away the fact that Mum was always there. We've spoken on the phone weekly since Dad died, and then almost daily this year. To lose such a companion is truly devastating.

Tonight I told Mum I was ready to let her die. I said it was the will of nature and I wasn't going to fight it.

She warned me that I must prepare myself to come in one morning and find her dead.

I told her I was ready.

Sunday 1 October 2006
Day nine of only water: four cups.

Sometimes my perceptions of Mary are quite damning. I wonder if she has similar ones of me. We all assume that other people encounter us the way we perceive ourselves; however, I imagine this concordance happens very rarely. She must think I am self-righteous and stubborn. I'm sure Fergus and Richard think I am over-casual to the point of being flippant. Of course none of them is right.

We all offer different faces to different people. With Mary I probably am more stubborn and sanctimonious, because by being so it allows me to restrain her when she is freewheeling on a destructive path. With Fergus and Richard, perhaps I do become flippant in an unconscious attempt to break the shackles of their rigid patterns of thought and behavior. But underneath there is the real me, the "me" that is perceived by me. Surely that is who I really am?

I wonder what self-image Mary has. Strong, confident, and in control? Not a chance; that is just her window display to the world. Maybe she sees herself as the victim or the fighter, because the odds have been stacked against her. I think I'm getting close.

And Fergus and Richard? They can be so damn conservative. Do they see that in themselves when they look in the mirror? No. They must see, "mature, sensible, responsible, and dependable."

This analysis wouldn't be complete without pondering Mum. Clearly my perception of her is a far cry from Jo's, which is different again from Mary's and Fergus's. Like the rest of us she has a different face for each of us, even though she may be in all our company at the same time.

How does she perceive herself? Now I am really going around in circles. I will pursue this line of thought another time.

During the night Mum fell off the commode and hit her head on a chair. This was when I left her alone once I had positioned her on it. She is now sporting a red bruise above her left eye. I told her that even I could see the red. However, by the time I woke her in the morning she said she was feeling fine, was in no pain, and felt no hunger. I insisted that she must be hungry. She was emphatic that she wasn't. I rearranged her bedroom furniture so she could prop herself up better when next using the commode.

We again talked about the survivors in a life raft and how she was outliving them, and rapidly catching up on Bobby Sands. She makes light of it, and ruefully suggests that she is immortal.

Mary has been here only a week and is about to leave. I am already feeling a weight off my shoulders. As soon as she got up she told me she was off back to Melbourne tomorrow as she had work to do and Mum could live a lot longer, although she also conceded Mum could die any day now. She said she had told Mum she was leaving, and that Mum told her that she was doing the right thing. I wasted no time in purchasing her ticket on the Internet.

I have to acknowledge that there are incredibly powerful emotions between Mum and Mary. It is easy for me to focus on my bond with Mum, but the bond between the two of them is very complicated. Mine is the simple love between a mother and son. Theirs is potent and complex. It seems to me that they are both seeking approval from each other and are both each other's harshest critics. I suspect that the cause of this complexity is something to do with Mum seeing Dad's characteristics in Mary. She responds to Mary as she did to him. I really don't understand what has happened between them and what is transpiring now. No, I don't envy her relationship with Mum at all. The sad thing is that many unresolved issues will probably remain.

When I spoke to Mum later, she said she was happy for Mary to go because she talks to her like a patient and not a mother – always talking at her and not to her. She is like the hospital staff who spoke to her in the same way.

Anyway Mary and I are not parting on bad terms. I accept she doesn't want to be here, and can see she doesn't need to be, either. Mum is very manageable now that she is confined to bed. Someone from the hospital comes each day to wash her. Mary said she will return immediately when Mum's condition becomes terminal. I'm not sure how she will know when that is.

Mary has certainly left the house in a far cleaner state than when she arrived. She is an incredible germ freak, spending every free moment polishing, scrubbing and vacuuming. In this one week she cleaned virtually every corner of the house. It drove me crazy! I always felt so uncomfortable and guilty with her vacuuming around my feet. My mind was so focused on Mum, I didn't have the desire to do housework. I don't think Mary wanted me to do my share. She claimed that she did this to stop herself from going insane with boredom. I suspect that one of us was going to lose it if she stayed any longer.

There seems to be a plateau in Mum's health. Dr. MacDonald was also very surprised at Mum's condition today as he is expecting her to go quickly. I previously gave her until next weekend when Fergus comes, but she may live longer. She is surviving by using up any fat and muscle on her body. It is just wasting away while her brain stays absolutely fine. All I can do is keep her in good spirits when she is awake (she dozes on and off most of the day now), and desperately hope I have no new crises to deal with.

Monday 2 October 2006
Day ten of only water: four cups.

It was an uneventful day today.

Mary's character is so dynamic that her departure has left a vacuum.

I wonder how much of an influence Dad had on shaping Mary's personality. Theirs was not a good relationship. The rest of us were intimidated by Dad's fierce, autocratic rule and we never contemplated standing up to him as Mary did. Looking back now, I can't help but admire her bravery in opposing a man whose judgment was questionable and whose discipline was total. Of course, the reason she stood up to him was that it was in her nature – she has a similar personality to Dad.

Such conflicts can leave scars.

In spite of my negative feelings for Mary, I acknowledge that I am feeling more negative about her now because I am under such stress. I really must not forget the glorious color she has brought to my life over the years. Even though she is five years older than me, our studies overlapped for several years as students at Otago University. We ended up socializing quite a bit considering our age gap, and we had a lot of memorable occasions together.

During this time I witnessed the early years of her relationship with Richard. Come to think of it, I also went on honeymoon with them around the Eastern Cape, after their wedding in Napier. It seems strange taking friends and family with you on honeymoon, but that was the generous spirit of Richard's family. Richard was besotted with Mary and could not see the warning signs of the suffering she would bring him later.

The Last Waltz: Love, Death & Betrayal

After they had children and moved to Hong Kong, I always enjoyed being an uncle to her three daughters. This included making several trips to visit them in Hong Kong, every year or two, en route to and from New Zealand. This kept our sibling relationship strong.

Mary has a dynamic personality and her presence fills a room as soon as she enters it. She always seems to have friends following her and unquestioningly doing things with her, at her command. I have also always noticed that other strong-minded women are drawn to her like a magnet.

Sadly the bottom line is that Mary is overbearing and manipulative, and her behavior is erratic. These traits combined with her high intellect make her a dangerous person to get too close to – if you threaten or challenge her she has a knack of embarrassing and humiliating you.

Tuesday 3 October 2006
Day eleven of only water: four cups.

After such a dramatic and stressful month this is the easiest time I have had with Mum because she is totally confined to her bed and I don't worry about her trying to do things on her own. After the last few months of an emotional rollercoaster ride, I have done all my grieving and we have said many goodbyes. It has taken her a while to let go of her independence, but now it's done we are both at peace. The main nursing duty for me is to lift her on to the commode twice a day and top up her water glass three times a day. That is why Mary left. She saw there was nothing else to do but wait and try to keep Mum from being unhappy.

Mary is in a better position than I am to gauge how long Mum has left. She thought Mum could still live for some time on water, although she said there was not much information to go on. I am worried about what will happen if one of her organs packs up. Surely her body can't just carry on functioning normally on water? Surely something will just fail completely? What will I do, since I have agreed to her request not to be taken to hospital again? I have promised to honor her Living Will. But what if she is in excruciating pain with a burst kidney? Will I leave her to die a tortured death? I need to apply my mind to this possibility now, rather than be faced with this dilemma in the middle of the night.

I spoke to the district nurse today about how long she thought Mum could live on water alone. She said she had no idea as it was almost unheard of for someone to take such drastic measures to kill themselves. She said the longest case they have on hospice records is a Chinese woman who survived for twenty-one days on water alone.

I told this to Mum. That was a big mistake as it genuinely upset her. All day she kept referring to this woman who had lived for twenty-one days. I tried to explain to her the irrelevance of this fact, because the survival time is dependent on the health of the individual. The Chinese woman could have had more fat, and her cancer could have been less advanced. But Mum would not listen to reason and kept saying she didn't want to live for so long. While I was reading in the living room I heard her on the phone to several people telling them about this. She was really in shock. Mum has now gone for ten days drinking only water. There is no way in the world she will break this record. It's strange how another eleven days seems like nothing to me, but to Mum it seems like eternity.

I am now reluctantly applying my mind as to what to do with the house. Fergus and Jo want it sold. Mary has asked if I could keep the house in the family with her. She wants us to raise a mortgage bond to buy out our siblings and use the rent money to cover it. It is a high risk venture, but a nice idea to keep the house in the family, while having a security net of property outside South Africa.

Wednesday 4 October 2006
Day twelve of only water: three cups.

Poor Truffle slept in the sun on the balcony today and refused to sleep on Mum's bed in protest at being kicked out last night! Truffle had better get used to it because she will be out every night now. Mum has lost the use of her legs and can't kick Truffle off her body when she gets too heavy. This caused Mum a lot of discomfort until I arrived in the morning to free her legs of Truffle's bulk.

The Last Waltz: Love, Death & Betrayal

Truffle is definitely putting on weight. I have been spoiling her with sachets of cordon bleu cat food. I've even been giving her dashes of cream in her milk saucer each morning, although Mum advised me against doing that. She says I am killing Truffle with too much love.

Since Mum still has movement in her arms, I have wrapped a cord around her knees that she can use to pull her legs up during the night when they get uncomfortable. It works well. She is now developing a bedsore on one side so I will have to start turning her every few hours. I am getting a sore back from leaning over the bed to pick her up. I am surprised at how heavy she is, although there is a steady deterioration in her health each day. I can't understand why such an intellectual person does not get bored, especially when she can no longer read, although this is relieved by listening to audio tapes.

The focal point of my anxiety each day is when I put Mum on the commode. This activity represents so much about the situation we find ourselves in. It is embarrassing and humiliating for Mum and it highlights her total dependency on me, and it is the most risky part of the day in terms of potential injury. The process is complicated by trying to preserve Mum's dignity as best I can. In the same motion of pulling down her blankets, I ensure her nightie has not crept up and exposed her body. I then lift her from the bed to the commode, which is a far from easy task. I respect her privacy by stepping into the living room and drawing the curtain between the rooms. I am only a meter or two away and can come quickly if she loses balance. I anticipate that it is only a matter of time before I will have to stand beside her and hold her. Mum dreads this routine because it is so exhausting for her. She gasps for breath at each step in the process. Once back on her bed, she gives a big sigh of relief that it is over.

Thursday 5 October 2006
Day thirteen of only water: four cups.

Gwyneth visited today. It was a balmy day and she went on a hunt around the garden for a flower that was mentioned in a

The Last Waltz: Love, Death & Betrayal

novel she was reading. Mum told her that she had them in her garden and Gwyneth became determined to find them. She must be in her seventies and is far from nimble, so she had to tread carefully through the lush undergrowth and around the maze of small shrubs and trees that make up Mum's wild garden.

Mum was enthusiastically negotiating her garden up to a couple of months ago. She always wore large black gumboots and would be up and down the garden, including the steep sloping wooden path leading up to her balcony, all with careless abandon. It was an unsettling sight for all of us, especially when the phone rang and she would make a desperate dash to the house.

Gwyneth wasn't able to find the flower she was looking for, even though Mum gave quite specific directions as to where it should be. Instead she returned to Mum's bedside with a delightful bouquet of mixed flowers and discussed each flower with her. This really made Mum's afternoon. After forty-five minutes Gwyneth had to rush off to a coffee appointment, having to leave seventeen minutes early because of the extra travelling time to get back to Dunedin. I am very impressed by Gwyneth's dedication to her ageing friends. There really are some wonderful angels around.

It gives me hope for us all.

As she was leaving I could see Gwyneth enjoyed discreetly looking around the walls and shelves of the house while she had the opportunity. She said she was surprised that there wasn't a photo of Dad hanging on any wall. I shrugged off this comment. She then said, "Your father certainly was a high achiever. Pat said he was medical superintendent of Seaview Hospital for seventeen years, a lieutenant in the New Zealand navy, and an officer in the British Army during the war. I would love to have met him. You must be so proud of him."

I agreed that he had achieved a lot.

Gwyneth continued, "I have met a number of people in medical circles who knew him and said he truly had the Irish 'gift of the gab' and was highly entertaining."

I told her I would dig up a photo of him for when she visited next week.

The Last Waltz: Love, Death & Betrayal

I didn't say that although the outside world loved Dad, they didn't have to live in the same house as him.

After she left I went and found a photo of Dad to show her next week. I didn't think it was my decision whether to hang it on the wall. Mum and Dad did not have a good relationship. It lacked all those ingredients that make a relationship work. We never saw any signs of warmth or affection between them. Not once did I see a kiss, a hug or any hint of love. All we saw was this total control and domination by Dad. He was constantly dishing out orders, often raising his voice if they were not acted on to his liking immediately. It was always worse when there was a special occasion like a birthday, Christmas, or a family dinner. On these occasions the house was a pressure cooker of tension until the drinks started to flow. And Mum wonders why I am still unmarried at forty-five.

It is now very late and I have just tucked Mum into bed. It takes a long time as her legs are totally immobile and I have to keep moving them until she thinks they will be comfortable for a few hours. I am frightened about the future and how I am going to get her on to the commode when she has no strength at all. I guess I will just have to find a solution to each problem as it arises.

Mum has been bedridden for nearly two weeks, so all the things I did with her I now do alone, from her complicated coffee preparation in the morning to lunch on the balcony, shopping in town, drives on the peninsula, cooking at night, and BBC dramas and documentaries in the evening. She now sleeps a lot and I have developed new routines.

Mum is getting sadder and sadder. She is living only on water but still wakes up every morning feeling fine. If I sit on the edge of her bed sipping my coffee for too long in the morning the conversation will eventually go to her agony of not dying and asking how she can speed up the process. On these occasions she constantly compares herself to lifeboat survivors and calculates that she can't have long to go. I spoke to Mary on the phone today and she thinks Mum's cancer has stopped spreading because she is not feeding it the food it needs to grow. This theory makes sense. At least she is not in cancer-induced pain. But how will she die now? Of malnutrition? How do people die of malnutrition? I am always asking the district nurses for advice but they can't tell me anything. This really is a case of the blind leading the blind.

Mum says she will hold on until Fergus gets here. I am not sure if she is consciously holding on or if she knows she has no choice. She keeps saying she is immortal. I am sure she says it to try to tempt fate to strike her down, but fate is not so kind to her.

The prospect of eternal life is the metaphysical holy grail of medicine, not to mention being the improvable premise on which most religions have been founded. Most people are so afraid of dying, but in reality the alternative is a far worse option.

Imagine if living forever was possible. Then the only way out would be suicide. But if suicide became the way to end life, then living forever would be a very sad prospect for humankind.

Richard from my Cape Town kitchen-bridge team often proudly proclaims his intention to live to one hundred and seventeen. What's the point? Our bodies keep aging. Hearing will go first, followed by eyesight, then the ability to walk. Do we want to be one hundred and seventeen, sitting in a wheel chair, deaf and blind – alive but certainly unable to play bridge?

Mum can't paint or read. How could she cope if she had to live for another thirty years?

I have decided not to speculate on when Mum might die. I can't be planning my life after she goes. It is better to believe that I will not be back in South Africa until the distant future, and just treasure my time with Mum as much as possible.

I am now in quite a different mental state than I was last month. I feel ready for Mum's death and realize that if it isn't soon she may end up with the undignified and ghastly death she so fears.

The Last Waltz: Love, Death & Betrayal

Friday 6 October 2006
Day fourteen of only water: four cups.

Another quiet day with Mum has passed. Once again, a couple of visitors popped by to chat to her. She really has some very loyal and devoted friends in Dunedin. They hold Mum in such regard. She is always very polite and dignified, even if she would prefer just to close her eyes and sleep. When she does want to sleep we have a code where I put my face close to hers to speak, so the visitors can't see her face and she can wink at me to
indicate she is going to pretend to sleep.

I am making my peace with Mary when she phones each day. She said it would be easy for her to feel jealous of my close bond with Mum, but that she couldn't feel anything negative about me when I had always been such a sweet brother. She added that I had never tried to keep Mum to myself but had encouraged her, Mary, to share the experience. She made an interesting observation that I see some truth in.

Mum had always been doted on by her father as a child, and throughout my life Mum has always said that I have a very similar personality to her father. It is now as if she is slipping more into her childhood and seeing me as a fatherly figure to take care of her.

Even if this is the case I am quite happy with that, as long as Mum is smiling and content.

One night when Mary went to arrange her sheets and blankets and tuck her in, she said she wanted me to do it because I knew exactly what to do! Of course anyone could tuck in blankets, but it did indicate some emotional dependency.

Verna also popped in to see her today as a friend, not as her home helper, and told me how Mum had been miserable before I came back to New Zealand and that she really picked up when she knew when I was coming.

This confirms to me the importance of my staying here.

Mum has told me several times that I should go and buy myself the jersey she liked from the sheep farm on the peninsula where we bought the first one. She said I am always wearing the same one and it looks as if I have only one jersey.

Anyway, a few days ago I did visit the farm and bought the plain grey jersey she liked without telling her. When I wore it this morning she immediately noticed and casually said, "I like your jersey!"

She notices more and more the things that would normally pass her by.

Recently I was wearing a blue T-shirt instead of the usual white ones, and she commented that she liked this one because white T-shirts look more like underwear.

On another occasion she commented on a Calvin Klein logo on a shirt I was wearing, and said she thought it such a waste of money buying clothes that had fashion logos on them.

She was impressed though when I told her I had got it second-hand.

The funny thing is that in all my life Mum has never until now commented on any clothes I have worn.

Saturday 7 October 2006
Day fifteen of only water: four cups.

John Francis phoned early to say he couldn't visit this weekend since he didn't have any petrol, but was sure he could come early next week. Jonah then phoned to say she didn't think she could make it tomorrow night because it would be high tide. Later Richard phoned to say he was "Either" coming for lunch "Or" he would pop by during the evening, depending on some complicated circumstances which I lost track of. I told him I would prefer to know when he was coming so I could plan my day. He said in that case he would visit in the evening. Since Richard wasn't coming during the day I made only a quick trip into town to do the shopping. I didn't have time to swim as I didn't want to leave Mum alone for so long. When I got back at lunchtime Richard was there with a female friend and one of his daughters. I was far from happy. If I had known he was coming at lunchtime I would have stayed in town for a much-needed swim. Richard could see my frustration. I guess I have no right to be angry. I should be grateful for any help. It is just so frustrating that he can't be more decisive about his plans.

Richard stayed for a couple of hours, sitting on the balcony with his friend. I had a sleep in my room. I had no desire to play host. I was worried that Mum would be upset. She is lying in bed waiting to die, while able to see people on her balcony enjoying wine in the sun.

Of course there is no reason why these people should not continue to enjoy life, but perhaps it is bad taste doing so in front of Mum, as if she no longer existed. I know how upset she was when Nina and I sat on the balcony drinking coffee in her field of view.

There must be times when she feels her world is being taken away from her.

Perhaps I am being over-sensitive.

This afternoon Peter Hinds visited. I have spoken to him a number of times in the garden now. He seems to be the only person who genuinely condones someone ending their life prematurely if they are suffering in the terminal stages of illness. He knows Mum wants out of this life, and in some ways I think that is why he keeps visiting. It's as if he wants to be there, if needed.

Today I decided to try out one of Mum's morphine tablets. I've been collecting her
weekly prescription. Mum wants to make sure she has a good supply. Not until today did I know what effect they have. But oh boy, it was good! Mum is in for a treat.

After Richard left I took a tablet on an empty stomach with a big glass of water. I went for a walk up the hill, as I thought that these conditions should all maximize the effect. Initially I noticed nothing. After about half an hour or so, when I was thinking this drug was a big myth, I started feeling the euphoria and it was amazing. The walk back seemed to last forever as my brain had sped up faster than normal time. I can understand how weak people can so easily get hooked.

The reason I tried the morphine was to follow a medical practice that Mum had developed. She told me many years ago that before she prescribed some new medication she would test it on herself first. She simply wanted to be sure of whatever she was prescribing.

She claimed on occasions the medications she gave to her outpatients were sugar candies: she dished these out in cases where her patients didn't need anything except the psychological benefit of taking medication.

In the evening, when the morphine had worn off, I told Mum that I had tested one of her tablets. She was alarmed, saying, "You mustn't do that."

I replied, "I only did what you did when you prescribed new medication."

I was surprised by her reply: "I don't want you to waste them. I may need every pill you have."

Mum was not at all concerned that I had tried morphine. Rather it was the loss of one of her tablets. I calmed her by telling her that she had a big supply and that it was growing by the week. Her eyes lit up and she asked how many she would need. I said I didn't know, but that she shouldn't think about it – Fergus was on his way to say goodbye to her. She then commented that this was not the kind of thing Fergus should know about. I don't know why Mum protects Fergus's innocence so much when he is quite a big boy at fifty-five.

Mum then said to me, "You are not happy." I replied that of course I was not happy watching her die. She said, "No, it's more than that." I reminded her that I am an optimistic person. She said, "You are happy on the surface, but you carry the cares of the world on your shoulders. You are the same as my father."

No. I can manage to carry only the cares of my mother. Perhaps she is just wondering why I took the morphine.

Sunday 8 October 2006
Day sixteen of only water: three cups.

My life with Mum is full of circles. We have daily circles and weekly circles and circles within circles. But running through these is a thick bold straight line: this is the line of Mum's life, which will end when she stops breathing. As each day passes, the intensity of the circles is becoming weaker as the straight line becomes increasingly bold.

The variations in the daily routines are becoming fewer. In the morning I get up and move quietly into the living room, gently drawing the curtain open to reveal her harbor view. I then tiptoe into her room and check that she is okay.

Yet the pattern is different now. As I draw open the curtain I take a deep breath, to prepare myself for what may await me as I turn to look at Mum. Each day, as I turn around, I tell myself that Mum is dead, to prepare myself.

Today was even more different. As I drew open the curtain and turned toward Mum's room and saw her still head on the pillow, and motionless body, I said to myself, "Now is the day. Please be dead." It seems so heartless but I know she is going to be gone one morning; and today I felt I was strong enough to take it. She wasn't dead. She opened her eyes and asked, Did Norton say if he was bringing a muesli bar today?

I felt huge relief.

Each passing day Mum gets a little worse and gives up a little independence to me. The procedure we have to go through when using the commode is getting more complicated. I wish she would stop wearing panties. Perhaps she feels that they symbolize the last threads of her tattered dignity.

A new problem has emerged, in that her bedsores are starting to hurt. I now have to regularly move her legs and twist her hips. Unfortunately this also has to be done at least twice during the night, which is exhausting as it is so difficult to get back to sleep after each trip to assist her. I try to make it a pleasurable thing for Mum, and make a joke of moving her legs this way and that, trying to find a position that is comfortable for her.

She still keeps looking at her watch, wishing the time would speed up. I told her that it wouldn't make any difference since the time to her death was not predetermined. An interesting discussion about time ensued, which is one of her pet physics subjects. There is most definitely nothing wrong with her brain.

The Last Waltz: Love, Death & Betrayal

John Francis was able to pop in today after all. He came in with a sketch of a school he had done on the drive out here. I couldn't see the school, nor for that matter could I distinguish any man-made building.

Today Ian made his first visit to the house since I have been in the country. He has been putting it off week after week. He said he hates visiting people in Mum's condition because he never knows what to say. I kept telling him that the longer he left it the harder it would be. He should have come here in my first few weeks in the country. Even then, though, he would have felt uncomfortable about what to say to someone who was approaching death. As luck would have it, just as Ian was running out of things to say to Mum, who should knock at the balcony door but Norton with a muesli bar in one hand and his painting in the other. Ian then discreetly disappeared to the kitchen, where the two of us spent the afternoon copying some of his New Zealand music CDs to add to my collection. New Zealand has some very gifted female singers: Anika Moa, Brooke Fraser and Bic Runga are my favorites. Anika Moa is a huge talent. Her voice is beautiful poetry in song and I am surprised she hasn't made it on the world stage.

I popped in to check on Mum and Norton. He was busy explaining the painting he had nearly finished, of Mum and me. I didn't need to be an art expert to observe that the resemblance to us was not particularly striking. I was surprised when he proudly announced that he is going to show it in an exhibition in Dunedin next week. He said he would put it on sale for $800! I think appreciation of art is a very personal thing. I secretly removed the muesli bar from Mum's bedside table and hid it in the kitchen. While I was making Norton coffee, I noticed Ian devouring it. When I gave Ian a cup of coffee he was quite upset that I put full-cream milk in it. He was also emphatic that he takes no sugar in his coffee. This was quite surprising considering the thick sediment I found when washing his cup after he'd left.

I've been putting some thought into Mum's comment yesterday. Tonight I suggested to her that the reason she thinks I am unhappy is because I am not married with children. I told her that this is a very old-fashioned way of thinking in today's world, where busy social lives have become the replacement for families. I said I couldn't understand why people stayed together when they didn't make each other happy. This was not a good argument for someone of Mum's generation, where a couple stay together for life.

I reminded her that I was now forty-five, the same age at which her own father married for the first time. I reassured her that I was planning to have a family. Perhaps I would have told her this even if I wasn't, so as to let her go without having to worry about me. She was also probably thinking the same thing.

Monday 9 October 2006
Day seventeen of only water: two and a half cups.

I got very little sleep last night – somewhere between three and four hours. So tonight will have to be a Mogadon night. My mind is on high alert and prevents me from relaxing enough to doze off each time I return to my pillow. I will also try Valium, which should do the trick.

It must be in the genes that I like constant background music, since Mum is the same. It has been my job to make sure she has a constant supply of music or voices. In the daytime she prefers voices, so I either have the radio on or I play one of the Somerset Maugham *Of Human Bondage* audiotapes. I am getting quite engrossed in this story as I often sit and listen to it with Mum. Sometimes she falls asleep during the tape, so when later in the day she wants the tape put on again, I replay the same section without telling her. There are only thirty-four tapes so I don't want them running out (she is up to tape seventeen). She is quite hooked on the articulate voices.

This morning when I popped in to check on her about 6am her radio was off, which concerned me. I gently woke her and asked why. She explained that she had turned it off because there was a news story about airlines on, and she never listens to anything about airplanes when her children are flying. Fergus will be leaving for New Zealand soon, and Mum once again fears a major air disaster. I tried to convince

The Last Waltz: Love, Death & Betrayal

her that statistics had been published showing that you are more likely to die from a bee-sting or falling down a manhole in the street, than an airplane crash.

There was another new sign of decline today. She has got to the point where she is struggling to hold the glass to drink her water. This is a critical turning point that we discussed some weeks ago, as it means that she may no longer be able to take an overdose by herself. Her intention was to overdose on her own if the need arose, and if she got to this stage she had gone too far and would be in an "undignified decline." Well, I think it's happening now.

I can only hope Mum is getting enough enjoyment out of life to want to keep living. Her eyes certainly lit up when I presented her with a tiny glass of freshly squeezed orange juice this morning. I promised her I would give it to her only this once. It is not as if it has many calories, and would give her a small pleasure in life. She had one token sip and said it tasted wonderful. She may have only pretended to take it, so as not to offend me.

We try to make it fun when I turn her every few hours. As I move her legs, knees and feet, she gives me a running commentary of instructions: "The left knee up a bit, right foot straighter, left knee over right knee, no, too much right leg, back a bit."

I told her we are finished with the ballroom dancing and are now "Doing the Hokey Cokey." This afternoon, when we had gone around in circles for some minutes trying to find a comfortable position for her legs, and no position seemed to be working, she gave a cheeky smile. She is still capable of teasing.

Tuesday 10 October 2006
Day eighteen of only water: two and a half cups.

I met Fergus at the airport this afternoon. I didn't think he would arrive in time to see Mum alive and I am very happy that Mum can say goodbye to all her children. Fergus and Mum have a shared interest in the environment, science and global politics, but never anything personal. They are both very conservative and have very traditional values. It is

The Last Waltz: Love, Death & Betrayal

appropriate that Fergus becomes the next family monarch. He has no animosity towards any of his siblings, and we all have total respect for him.

He arrived after a very long flight that deviated from the direct route. Fergus is very reactionary and no matter how many times I have tried to lead him towards a more modern way of booking tickets through the Internet, he insists on walking down to his local travel agent in South Wimbledon and doing it the hard way, just as it has been done in England for decades.

Fergus came through the arrival gate wearing the same colorless clothes he has worn for most of his life: loose-fitting brown corduroy trousers, a checked shirt, a grey cardigan, and brownish slip-on shoes. He looks as if his mother dressed him. He has such an extraordinary wit and unique angles on most topics of conversation, but this doesn't come across in his clothes. So he is not the type of guy you are likely to seek out to talk to, yet you must do so to discover his fascinating personality. In spite of his present image, Fergus has certainly been popular with the ladies. I have recently been going through photos of him as a young man, photos that show a very trendy, good-looking Fonz-type character with dark, swept-back hair, beer in one hand, often leaning on a large American automobile with a good-looking "chick" close by.

Fergus and I have totally different personalities but there are extraordinary coincidences in our lives, even though they have hardly overlapped as he left home when I was eight. We both regularly play tennis, bridge and chess, and he enjoys saroc dancing while I dance ballroom and Latin. We also both have Ph.Ds. in microbiology and have specialized in genetics. I can't think of an explanation for these similarities. The good thing about our shared interests is that we always have something to bind our friendship, which helps, since I am not so inclined to drinking in pubs. It interests me, too, that Fergus and I have also never been married.

Anyway, Fergus is here now and I am very happy to have his stabilizing influence, though I'm not sure how much help he will be since he leaves in twelve days and will need some nights to get over jet lag. He is also a little squeamish, so I

The Last Waltz: Love, Death & Betrayal

can't imagine his being comfortable doing what I've been doing.

Fergus was very disappointed at the weather that greeted him. Snow is falling over almost the whole country including Dunedin (he was really hoping to go back to London sporting a suntan). He was surprised by Mum, who was healthier than he'd expected after all the horror stories he'd heard. He reprimanded her for going on her hunger strike and said it was not the way to die.

Fergus had an early night as he'd certainly had a marathon journey.

After he had gone to bed, Mum and I had a morphine party. She was keen to experience for herself the euphoria that I had described. I said it was a good idea to try one now, so she knew what to expect in case she needed to take them regularly.

We followed the same sequence we do with Mogadons. We lined up the tablets and discussed whether they should be broken into pieces so we could slightly increase or decrease her dosage next time. Unlike Mogadons, these tablets were not so easy to break into pieces, but I could cut them in half. We took one and a half each with a glass of water. I gave Dad's traditional "Davison toast" to create a jovial atmosphere. When I damned the Pope, Mum said he had already damned himself today with his derogatory comment about Muslims. I agreed, adding that his comments could be the catalyst for a holy war. I asked if she minded not being around to find out.

The answer was of course "No!"

In any other context, it would be pretty unusual to be getting high on morphine with your Mum. It's funny how life works out. It was Mum who actually encouraged me to take one with her. I guess it was like sharing coffee in the morning: it was more sociable for her to share the experience than do it alone. She also knows how responsible I am and that I would never abuse such a drug.

In hindsight it would have been better for me not to have one so I could monitor the effect on her, because it appeared to bring about little or no change. Perhaps it made her more relaxed, but it certainly didn't have the euphoric effect that it had on me. I spent an hour or so entertaining Mum with some dance steps. I had to use Truffle as a partner at times.

Mum stopped me when I thought of wrapping up a tiny piece of morphine in some cat meat. Truffle loved all the attention and showed her appreciation by dribbling on Mum all evening. It is now after 2am. I had better get some sleep in case Fergus wants to play tennis in the morning. He has brought his racquet from London, so he is taking me as a serious threat.

Wednesday 11 October 2006
Day nineteen of only water: two cups.

I had a disturbed night after our party. Firstly Mum needed to go to the toilet at 4am but I didn't hear her bell. Fortunately, Fergus heard it as he was up himself. I put her on the commode, though as it turned out she didn't really need to go. She was just scared of having an accident when Fergus was here and thought she would try anyway. Then we didn't hear her bell ringing continuously from 6am until I surfaced after 7am. She was lying on a bed sore and was in agony. Consequently she is very tired today. I am exhausted as I am getting no more than four hours' sleep each night. I just can't relax, and the less I relax the less sleep I get. I feel in a different world.

When Fergus got here Mum was at her best. He considered her intellect and personality unchanged. Today, however, we can see a marked decline. She even seems a little confused. When Fergus and I returned after four hours of playing tennis and shopping, she went on and on about how miserable she had been and how much pain and suffering she'd had while we were out. She said she was in such discomfort that she considered dropping off her bed and dragging herself to the couch (probably impossible now).

I had never seen this behavior before and put it down to her emotional dependency on me: for Fergus to take me away for such a long time was almost an act of betrayal. She was jealous and didn't want to share me with anyone. This was also like when she asked Jo to go back home after a few days here, and when she told Mary to let me tuck her into bed.

More and more I realize how fleeting life is. I look at this house full of Mum's presence, all the things she has made and painted, and all her books and arty things. These are nothing without her. They exist as they are only while she is alive. I realize more and more how unimportant possessions are.

Fergus and I think she has only a few more days left to live, but I have no knowledge of how long the human body can keep going on water. She still keeps wishing to be dead, so it is not willpower that's keeping her alive, but rather the simple biology of a human heart that won't stop beating. Today's indication of her decline was that for the first time she did not want the radio, CD, or audio book on. I have asked her several times if I can play something and each time she says no. She is also sleeping much more, and when she is awake I ask her what she is thinking about and she is unable to remember. I was always asking her questions to keep her mind alert, but now she has asked me not to as it is too difficult and taxing for her to think of the answer, although Fergus asked her what the capital of Mongolia was, and she got it right. (I didn't have a clue.)

I wonder how much yesterday's morphine is still acting on her brain. It didn't seem to be affecting her last night. Perhaps she has a much slower metabolism than I do. It does seem to take longer to affect her than it does me. Incidentally, last night's morphine had no obvious effect on my tennis abilities today (although Fergus was very jetlagged).

Thursday 12 October 2006
Day twenty of only water: two cups.

For two months now, I have been in a state of high alert every night. Last night I went to bed and told myself to switch off and let Fergus be on guard for Mum's bell, yet I still had a bad sleep.

I totally misread Mum's condition yesterday. Today she is back to what has been her normal self. She correctly answered general knowledge questions that she couldn't answer yesterday. She asked for her radio or audio book to be on all day, and she is a lot less sleepy. The reason for yesterday's disorientation had to have been the morphine the previous night. Perhaps I gave her too much. I am certain it is very slow acting on her. There is no need to give her more until she is in pain.

Today, considering her lucid state, I asked her which she wanted: morphine and to be disconnected or no morphine and be depressed about not dying. She told me that I must decide as she doesn't want to make any more decisions. I told her that she was leaving me the impossible choice of giving her morphine and effectively losing my mother, or keeping an anxious, unhappy one.

She was still adamant it was my decision. Doctors are no longer involved now, so it really is my call.

Fergus cannot stay long because he has only a small amount of leave from work. He can't wait for Mum to die since no one can say how long she has. I told Mum that she has now broken the record of the Chinese woman. She looked at me in total disbelief and frustration and said, "I am immortal."

Gwyneth shows incredible commitment to honor every appointment. This morning the road to Dunedin was closed along the harbor because of damage caused by very high tides and she had to drive over the back hills to get here. These narrow, winding, high roads were very slow-moving due to the traffic that was now diverted on to them. When I phoned and suggested she cancel today she wouldn't hear of it, and made provisions for an extra fifty-five minutes' travelling time in her diary.

I showed Gwyneth a photo of Dad. He looked very handsome in his military uniform. He had a big smile, strong facial features, and was beaming with confidence and authority. I could see Mary in him.

I also showed Gwyneth a family photo. It was a formal portrait taken when I was about four. We looked like a model family, all smartly dressed, four happy children gathered around our proud parents. It all seemed so perfect then.

The Last Waltz: Love, Death & Betrayal

But look at what became of us. This time comes from that time. What was wrong then?

Gwyneth had brought the flower that she had been looking for in Mum's garden. She proudly gave it to Mum, with the story of how she got it.

I kindly asked Gwyneth not to come next week. I told her that although Mum appreciates her visitors it is becoming a huge strain for her to talk to them. Gwyneth understood and said she is amazed that Mum is still alive. She said she is always expecting my call with news of her death.

Friday 13 October 2006
Day twenty-one of only water: two cups.

What an extraordinary night last night. Fergus had gone out drinking with Richard, and I was going through Mum's drawers and came across a pile of unused diaries she was given by medical reps when she worked. She used them for scrap paper. I flicked through each one before I tossed them in the fire, and then, to my astonishment, in one book was written a personal diary. I couldn't believe Mum had one. She usually kept her emotions to herself. But here I was reading her personal feelings being expressed in this very risky form, in her doctor's scrawled handwriting.

After I had browsed through it I went into her room and turned off her audio-book to get her attention. She slowly opened her eyes and looked at me. I then asked if she ever kept a diary. She was very used to my daily barrage of questions, traps and riddles and whispered, "No," in the dejected voice of someone uninterested in life. I told her I had just gone through her stuff and found one. She looked startled, lifted her head, and opened her eyes wide, exclaiming, "What!" I felt I had brought her back from the dead!

I opened her diary and randomly read a line dated 1979: "Took Jo to Dunedin. She had just got the dole. She bought a lacy dress and a shawl." Mum became quite interested and said she remembered this and completed the rest of the story in detail, which I confirmed by further reading.

The Last Waltz: Love, Death & Betrayal

I then chose another seemingly meaningless line from a different page: "The white line zone is for loading and unloading only, no parking."

Mum immediately said, "Yes, that was when we went to Los Angeles." Sure enough, when I turned to the previous page I saw that this was during our trip to Los Angeles twenty-seven years ago to meet up with Fergus, Mary, and her boyfriend at the time.

Mum said that the diary had to be destroyed since there were some things that should not be seen. She was so wide-awake and receptive now. We could have been having this discussion twenty years ago.

When Fergus came home he was anxious to know whether he featured in the diary. I thought it best to tell him that he didn't. Perhaps I should have told the truth as maybe he is offended that he didn't feature in Mum's private thoughts. It's hard to gauge how sensitive Fergus is. Like Mum, he keeps his emotions to himself. I wonder if he keeps a diary.

The three of us then chatted for a while. Fergus is always good-humored and relaxed after he's had a drink. We discussed the PIN number for Mum's EFTPOS debit card. I wanted Fergus to hear the story from Mum's lips of how I worked out her number. I had already told Fergus, but it was so incredible I wanted him to have confirmation of its authenticity while Mum was alive.

It happened shortly after I arrived and Mum wanted to give me a check to cover living expenses while I was here, since I had to do all the shopping. I said it would be easier just to let me use her debit card. She said she couldn't do that because the number was a secret and she wanted to take it to her grave.

She then went on to describe how incredible it was that no one could know her number, not even the bank. Even as a physicist, this concept was a bit confounding for her since she felt the number had to be somewhere.

I then asked her to let me work out the number. I took a stab and asked if it was to do with her father's birth date. She said no. I then asked if it was connected to her mother's birth date; she said not.

I said, "Is the number xxxx?"
Her eyes nearly popped out!
The number was correct!

She said I could use the card and I must never tell anyone the number.

Fergus and I then pondered how incredible it was that I could get a number that she had never written down or told anyone. Mum deduced that because she used this number each day she had somehow provided a mental link for it to get to my brain.

After Fergus had analyzed all this, he wanted to know whether this was a random number or did it have some link that would increase the chances of my getting it right. Mum volunteered the information that it was connected to our step-grandfather. I added an extra clue, which I'm sure was crossing Fergus's mind, by saying that it was not linked to his birth.

I did not get a lot of sleep because I took the liberty of reading Mum's diary. That was a privilege. The most enlightening thing from the night was to discover how attentive Mum is, especially having the ability to recall events from more than twenty-seven years ago from a single sentence.

Saturday 14 October 2006
Day twenty-two of only water: one cup.

This morning when I was turning Mum she said to me, "You didn't destroy my diaries as I asked, did you?"

"No," I replied.

Today Mum wanted to monitor the effects of another morphine tablet on her, so I gave her one early in the morning. By tonight I had lost her, in exchange for a pitiful child. Fergus and I went out for a drink with Richard, and arranged for Jonah to sit with her. Before we left, Morphine-Mum was saying to me that I couldn't stay away for too long as she would be in pain and misery. There was no logic in this, since there was nothing that Jonah couldn't do that I could, and she had not been in pain all day. At one point in the evening I phoned Jonah and she said Mum was constantly looking at her watch and asking when we would be back. I asked her to give Mum the phone and I got the sob story: "I am feeling so uncomfortable. Lots of pain and misery. When are you coming back?" I told her in an hour. She replied, "No, an hour is so long. Please come back now." I was hesitant. We were listening to Anika Moa giving a pub concert. However, we decided to go along with Mum and head back. Sure enough, I got the same complaint when I got back home about how miserable she had been (this is in front of poor Jonah, who had done such a great job).

I told Mum I would never leave her alone in the evenings again, which seems to be her worst fear. I guess her dependency is a natural consequence of having me nurse her through the last couple of months. Now there are childlike scenes when I disappear for too long, although morphine may be a factor.

Sunday 15 October 2006
Day twenty-three of only water: one cup.

This morning I put Mum's absurd logic from last night to her, and asked why it mattered my not being there when Jonah was doing the same things. She said she couldn't answer that but it did make a difference. I am now certain that the morphine is very slow acting on her. In fact, I am convinced that the greatest effect of the morphine is many hours later, as it seems to have little effect immediately after she takes it. She is completely normal tonight and has no recollection of her behavior yesterday. It is tricky dealing with two people now.

I am getting so confused. I am never sure what I have already written in this diary. There is a lot of repetition of thoughts and ideas in my head. It is just very therapeutic for me to keep writing in order to rationalize my emotions and what is happening each day. It is a relief having Mum back, out of the world of morphine. She is also showing concern about me and how I am holding up, which shows she is still my mother. I really am solely responsible for deciding which world Mum should be in; the real one as my mother, or the confused, childlike world of morphine. It's a tough decision. I think it is going to be forced on me, as she seems to be aching all over, not from cancer, but from lying so motionless all day.

In her awake state today she again categorically said that she can't continue in this misery and wants to end it. Her problem now is that it is very difficult for her to swallow pills, and she would need to swallow a lot of morphine tablets to be sure of dying. Time could be running out for her to do this unassisted. It still crosses my mind that she may not really have the willpower to end her life. Weeks ago she told me that she would do it after saying goodbye to Jo and Mary, and that she wouldn't wait for Fergus. Yet after Jo and Mary left she said she would hold on for Fergus. Then yesterday, she said it would be unfair to do it when Fergus was here as he didn't have the stomach for it. Fergus leaves in a week and this gives her reason to wait. Although when I told her Fergus would be here for a whole week she was totally taken aback, as she'd thought he was leaving much sooner. At least there are enough reasons to justify her wanting to continue.

Does she really want to die?

I think of how, when I go to the outdoor pool at the end of the summer season, the water is getting quite cold, but I know I will not leave until I have got into the pool. I will then procrastinate for a very long time before finally taking the plunge. No matter how long I delay that plunge it is always going to happen. Logically there is no reason to delay the inevitable, but I still do. It is the same when you are at death's door and you know the inevitable is waiting for you, but to plunge into that cold uncertainty is far from instinctive? Mum keeps holding on to life as much as she wants to let go of it.

How will it be to be dead?

Will we have that same relief as jumping into that cold pool at the summer's end? The fear of the cold water or the fear of death will have gone.

The real question is, how will it feel to have no fear? But there is no such thing as "no fear." It is impossible to imagine, like trying to imagine nothing.

The Last Waltz: Love, Death & Betrayal

Each one of us must confront these issues of death. Otherwise, we die never having contemplated the unknown that awaits us. I would prefer to die knowing that I didn't know.

The fact that Mum has been able to say goodbye to all her children is a wonderful thing. To her we represent her life. She loves us all, and she never doubts our love for her. To know that a child does not love you must be the greatest pain of all. I didn't love Dad. Jo doesn't love Mum. Dad didn't know it. Mum doesn't know it. Some things are better concealed.

All my life I remember Mum only ever having the one picture hanging on her bedroom wall. It was a photo of her father. It never crossed my mind to ask her about her love for him and how she felt when he died; she was twenty-eight. This photo still hangs on the wall at the end of her bed, as if he is still watching over her. Only now do I finally understand why. Tonight she asked me to put the photo on her bedside table so she could see it. I did this and also draped his Queen's Medal over it. Mum must have adored him so much, and must have been devastated when he died. Perhaps she knows the pain I face.

Monday 16 October 2006
Day twenty-four of only water: one cup.

It is a sad reality that Mum has planned her death very badly. She was so sure that starving herself was the only way to have some control over her destiny, but really this is the worst possible way to go. I think the rest of her life will not be very pretty.

Fergus is appalled at what Mum is doing to herself. He points out that if she had not chosen this absurd way to end her life she would quite likely be having a fairly enjoyable and worthwhile one. He also says that it is not too late for Mum to change her mind and end her life in a dignified manner.

While I was out swimming and shopping, Fergus was changing Mum's audio-book tapes at a fast rate. If you play one tape after another you can finish the book in a day, and this is what Fergus did. I had to convince Mum that Fergus got the numbering system wrong and put her back to tape twenty-four. She didn't seem to notice, as she was probably dozing through most of it.

Tuesday 17 October 2006
Day twenty-five of water only: one cup.

I met the pharmacist today. He knows Mum well and saw me with her many times over her last few visits. He must also have noticed that I have been coming in alone on the last few occasions to collect the morphine prescription. He hardly needed to be a rocket scientist to realize that Mum was nearing the end. Today I asked if I could speak with him alone.

He escorted me to a private office where I put my simple question to him: "How much morphine is a lethal overdose?"

He was a kind man with a gentle demeanor and showed no surprise or concern at my question. He initially said he didn't have any idea, and then told me to wait a few minutes. When he came back he said that he had looked up the highest recorded dose that someone had survived, and that it was one hundred and eighty milligrams.

Dr. MacDonald came to visit in the evening. He took Mum's blood pressure and pulse. As usual, Mum looked at him, anxiously awaiting the result. As usual, Dr. MacDonald said they were both normal. She was exasperated. She is desperate for her body to give up.

Every time Dr. MacDonald comes she tells him that she is going to drag herself down to the harbor at the end of her property and drown herself if he doesn't help her end her life. Dr. MacDonald always calmly tells her that this is not a good idea and that she is too weak to do it anyway.

Mum does seem dependent on his visits. It is as if she sees him as a confidante. She keeps up a normal facade with us, but as soon as Dr. MacDonald comes, she is brutal in her honesty of how she wants to die now. I always leave Dr. MacDonald alone with Mum, but of course I am listening around the corner, which he knows.

The Last Waltz: Love, Death & Betrayal

I can't really see the point of Dr. MacDonald's visits. He can't prescribe any medication since Mum won't accept anything. He can't do anything except have a chat. When we spoke tonight he again expressed his surprise that Mum was so strong, and still alive. She is down to only one glass of water per day. Now she is going to die of malnutrition, which she has proved is a very slow, miserable process.

The doctor and nurses are all guessing as to the future, and are all surprised she is still alive. We shouldn't really be surprised. Everyone who knows Mum says how stoic she is.

The irony of this terrible death is that if Mum had speculated a year ago about how she might die, she would have described her present predicament as the worst way to go. If she'd known this was going to happen she would certainly have chosen a different strategy. She is now just skin and bone.

And it is not over yet.

I just have to decide when and whether to start giving her morphine on a daily basis. Once she starts it she will be incapable of making any further requests or decisions, including whether to take an overdose. It will be wholly up to me, and I am certainly not going to murder my Mum.

Fergus is still here for a few more days, and it is good having him take night duty every second night, but even on my nights off I still can't sleep as my mind stays active just in case Fergus doesn't wake up to Mum ringing the bell.

The nursing role does not come easily for Fergus. She has certainly put him through the hoops on some nights, with lots of bell ringing, followed by lots of maneuvering of her legs. We speculate that she misbehaves more on Fergus's nights because it is a way of saying that she prefers me to assist her.

Our exhaustion is becoming evident in our tennis matches. At least Fergus's blister does not seem to be troubling him too much.

Tonight we will get a little respite since the hospice will be sending a nurse to sit with Mum all night. Apparently the nurse is not allowed to sleep, as she is a paid night nurse.

The purpose of these visits is to help the family of terminal patients get some quality sleep, rather than making any big difference to the patient. We are allowed seven nights per month, so I don't want to use them up too soon. I hope Mum doesn't mind a stranger.

Snow was falling on Mum's balcony at lunchtime, although the temperature got up to the low 40s during the day, with the same forecast for tomorrow.

Wednesday 18 October 2006
Day twenty-six of only water: one cup.

Belinda, the nurse, left early in the morning and left us a note detailing each hour of the night. At the bottom of the note she wrote, "PS: Who left the toilet seat up?"

I showed this to Fergus and he said, "But that's what blokes do, isn't it?"

Mum was very happy with Belinda. She is very kind and understanding, and granted Mum's every request without question. Once again I didn't sleep because I was concerned about a stranger looking after Mum. I had to check during the night to make sure she was okay, which incidentally defeats the whole purpose of a night nurse. Belinda said it is completely normal for the family not to sleep on the first night she stays, but then they get used to it. She is going to come again tonight so Fergus and I can get some good rest. Since there are two of us nursing Mum, we don't absolutely need her.

Fergus seems quite impressed with the nursing skills I have developed. I have often told him that I need all the practice I can get because, since I am younger, it is only a matter of time before I will be bathing him and putting him on a commode. I also suggested he start working on his fox trots and tangos.

Mum has been serene and smiling today. We had lots of chats and she showed her undiminished mental prowess. It is amazing that her body has wasted away to skin and bones yet the brain remains virtually unchanged. This is a clever feat of evolution, as surely the brain is the most important organ in the body. I keep wondering why another organ hasn't given up under this duress. Perhaps I have a nasty surprise still to come. I hope not, as I am too exhausted to deal with any more shocks. I don't seem to think very clearly these days.

The Last Waltz: Love, Death & Betrayal

We are making using the commode a more pleasurable routine. I sit her up in bed, and hold her for a minute or two for her blood pressure to adjust before lifting her. During this time I hold her with a two-arm hug to keep her balance, while sitting on the edge of the bed.

I discussed with the nurses today about giving Mum a catheter. I was very surprised that Mum agreed to this procedure, and the nurses inserted one.

This afternoon when Dr. MacDonald arrived I announced him: "Dr. MacDonald has come to make your day, Mum."

Her face lit up, showing exaggerated joy. "That's wonderful, wonderful."

I couldn't believe the pleasure in her eyes, so I asked her why she was so excited when he has come to see her so often. She replied, "Didn't you just say that Dr. MacDonald has come to end my days?"

"No, Mum, he's come to make your day."

Her smile faded, but she appreciated the funny side of it.

Mum speaks very little now, so I treasure every word. It's as if she is lying there cursing the fact that she can't die. She is looking so very frail. I feel I should stop all visitors soon.

I sat with her reading tonight. It was quite late when I said goodnight.

"What's the time, please?"

"It's nearly midnight, Mum."

"Oh good."

It's as if time is the only thing that's changing.

Thursday 19 October 2006
Day twenty-seven of only water: one cup.

I had another of those dreadful moments this morning. Mum was not at all happy with the catheter and she kept saying that she wanted to go on the toilet. I told her it was impossible, so her desire was in her imagination. She then said that she wanted it taken out. I said I would arrange it if she first relaxed and tried to let it do its job. Eventually she did this, but then insisted she had wet her mattress. Eventually I checked to make her feel better, and sure enough she was right – something had gone terribly wrong

The Last Waltz: Love, Death & Betrayal

with the catheter. This was extremely upsetting for her, although at this stage I think she feels no humiliation about anything. Life is becoming a struggle from one moment to the next.

I was trying to keep Mum on her mattress until the district nurses came, but eventually Mum wanted to go again. I wasn't going to disagree this time. I lifted her from the bed and was trying to put her on to the commode when there seemed to be something attached to her, holding her to the bed. Thinking it was just a sheet, I pulled her away from the bed. To my horror, I discovered that the catheter was attached by safety pins to the mattress and I was tugging at it. She gave a loud shriek in pain.

We were stuck as Mum's foot was now hooked on the side arm of the commode, and she was attached to the bed by the tube. I was losing grip of her in this trapped position and she was slipping from my grasp. I had to make an instant decision and instinctively pushed her towards the bed. Her knee made a cracking sound as it unhooked from the commode, she banged her head on the floor, and the catheter was pulled out.

Fergus had put his gumboots on and was nowhere within call. Poor Fergus. Although he is a dedicated man of duty, he would be much happier visiting Mum in a hospice with nurses doing all these messy personal things.

I untangled the knot of limbs and tubes, sheets and safety pins, and gently rested Mum on the bed to catch her breath. She seemed surprisingly composed after such an ordeal.

It took some time to tidy up. I realized I hadn't put Mum's hat back on, and apologized as I did so. She replied, "It doesn't matter. You've seen my bald head so many times before." This was sort of funny. I was trying so hard to maintain her dignity over what was such a small thing as seeing her bald head, while everything else was collapsing around us. It seemed like her final surrender.

The district nurses came to insert a new catheter at lunchtime. End of story? No such luck. Tonight she asked to go to the loo. Again I said it was impossible. She insisted, so I put her on the commode (after unpinning the catheter from her bed). Unbelievably she was able to. This should not be possible. I immediately phoned the doctor. He told me I must reinsert it, and gave me careful instructions.

This is getting out of control. There is no way in the world a son should have to do this.

I don't want any more crises like this one. I am too exhausted to deal with them. I get the awful feeling that this may only be the beginning.

Friday 20 October 2006
Day twenty-eight of only water: one cup.

Mum has made two bad decisions that have made this so much worse than it should have been. First, going on this starvation diet, and secondly, refusing to go into a hospice at this last hurdle.

Mum has said all along that she hates being her own doctor, and that she was forced to be until recently. I think she certainly took matters into her own hands when she began this diet, however. She has lived her life making decisions and that is the way it has ended. I suppose she should be commended for that. But now the time has come for me to decide.

The cheerless news continues. Mum is now experiencing real pain all over her body as opposed to discomfort. The district nurses were very concerned to learn today that she was not on morphine, even though I said she had turned it down each day I had offered it. I also told them how confused morphine made her and how it upset me. They reprimanded me, saying that my sole concern was her comfort (as if I didn't know that).

It has occurred to me that perhaps the constant discomfort she has been in over the last couple of weeks is the type of pain that morphine is prescribed for. Mum and I assumed the morphine was for some even worse pain that is still to come.

Perhaps she has been suffering unnecessarily.

Tonight I will start the morphine and assess its impact. I know that since I am starting it because of the pain, there will be no reason to stop it. This is in effect the last day I have my mother. I have made the decision while Fergus is here and in

The Last Waltz: Love, Death & Betrayal

agreement so I won't question later whether I decided this unilaterally and in a confused state.

Later the same day

I have just told Mum that I am going to have to put her on a daily dose of morphine. She didn't seem to mind, but she doesn't realize the effect morphine has on her, and the painful effect on her son, watching her slip into a confused fantasyland. I told her we must now say goodbye while she was still my mother. She said, "No goodbyes yet."

I replied, "No, Mum, this really is goodbye."

She didn't seem to mind but asked me to put some morphine tablets under her pillow, too. I felt she wanted the comfort of knowing they were there.

I took the opportunity to tell her that I would not be scared if she contacted me after she died. She smiled, indicating that she liked this idea, although I know she doesn't think it likely. I heard Fergus jokingly telling Mum that he didn't want her to come and spook him, even though he also has a lot of interest and theories on what happens after death. I would much rather be frightened and have a moment's insight, than not be, and live without that knowledge. There is a quote that has always stuck in my mind: a moment's insight is worth a lifetime's knowledge.

Mum is very familiar with my one experience with this sort of thing. This was after Dick Kammon died while out running. He was a professor of psychology at Otago University and Mary's boyfriend (he was lucky he didn't die many years earlier, since Dad always left a shotgun on the doorstep whenever he came to visit Mary in Hokitika).

Dick was an authority on parapsychology. He also knew about the death pact that Mum and I had, about contacting each other after death. He thought that was impossible. Anyway, I woke one morning with an overwhelming feeling that someone very close to me had just died, and was so concerned I spent the day checking that my immediate family were all accounted for. It wasn't such a surprise to learn that Dick had died. Who better to communicate with from his grave than a person he'd been carrying out parapsychology experiments with, and who had a death pact to expect communications from his mother when she died? This was my epiphany. I hope Mum can give me another message from beyond the grave. I am going to find out soon.

Mum wants to take an overdose, but with morphine in her system she can no longer give me a clear instruction. I cannot make the decision. I guess Mum and I will be in a state of limbo until her end and there will be little more to write about her.

Fergus leaves on Sunday, so I will be on night duty every night. I may put my mattress in her room. I am in such a state of exhaustion it will make no difference where my mattress is. I think my judgment is wavering, but I don't think I will have any more major decisions now. I will just wake and find Mum dead one morning.

This state of suspension could go on for some time. Mum had joked about doing a "Bobby Sands" – never really believing a starvation diet for her could get anywhere near to sixty-five days. Now she finds the joke not funny as she curses the fact that she appears to be immortal.

Later the same night

I have just given Mum the first of her tablets. I said goodbye to her as a mother. I also took a tablet myself, for strength.

Saturday 21 October 2006
Day twenty-nine of only water: one cup.

Today Mum was very confused under the influence of yesterday's morphine. She couldn't answer simple questions such as the capital of Brazil and Denmark, but this evening she was quite attentive. I said to her that Fergus was leaving tomorrow and she must say goodbye to him. I added that she would be saying goodbye forever. To my surprise she said, "Yes, it's very sad." She then told me to bring him in and she asked us to sit next to her. She began a speech in her faint voice that went something like this: "Fergus, you will now be in charge." Fergus and I looked at each other in surprise

The Last Waltz: Love, Death & Betrayal

because we had the impression that she had put me in charge. She then added, "You will be in charge of discipline, but I don't want you to be like Dad." Fergus and I again exchanged glances. But she was quite rational, continuing, "You boys can take the family silver. The girls already have most of the jewelry. I want you to put all of my small antiques on display in the kitchen for my friends to help themselves to the ones you children don't want." This all made sense as we had heard this request before. She then added, "I don't want there to be any arguing among you after I die." I told her that there would be no arguing and she replied, "Yes, you are all good children."

Fergus and I took the opportunity of Mum's lucidity to ask her questions about a few of her ornaments. We took each item to her and asked about its history. At one point I took in the pottery salt holder from the kitchen that I particularly liked. I asked, "Mum, did you make this?"

I was surprised by her reply, "I can't remember."

I persisted, "But you must know if you made it."

She replied, looking very guilty for not knowing, "I am really sorry, but I can't remember." She paused and added (perhaps to make me feel better), "I think I did." Mum taught us never to take credit for someone else's work, so I presume she made it. But it was sad she couldn't remember.

Mum was having a good evening and was speaking very intelligibly. She then asked Fergus to leave the room and proceeded to tell me that her life was so miserable she wanted to end it when Fergus left. A while ago she told me about a supply of amitriptyline which she had hidden. She said she found it in Dad's medical box after his death. Mum joked that it was his gift to her in case she had to end her own life if ever the circumstances arose. She now told me that it was concealed in a wooden box under the old grandfather clock in the hall. I immediately went and found it. I showed it to her. She said after Fergus leaves she will take her life. She seems to have forgotten about the morphine.

At the end of the night Mum wanted a hug and began singing a Robert Burns poem she knew from school:

The Last Waltz: Love, Death & Betrayal

"Ae fond kiss"
Ae fond kiss, and then we sever
Ae farewell, alas, forever
Deep in heart-wrung tears I'll pledge thee
Who shall say that fortune grieves him
While the star of hope she leaves him
Farewell, thou first and fairest
Farewell, thou best and dearest.

Mum was surprised I did not know this poem so I looked it up. When Fergus joined us we sang it together. It was a moving choice of verse.

Since Mum had had no morphine today and her mind was extraordinarily clear tonight, I quizzed her again on the capital of Denmark and Brazil, which she now knew. I recalled our conversations earlier in the day but she had no recollection. I told her how she had been insisting on using the toilet, in spite of having a catheter inserted, and again she had no idea.

I gave her a morphine tablet.

Sunday 22 October 2006
Day thirty of only water: one cup.

I took Fergus to the airport this morning. Before we left, I said I would leave him alone to say goodbye to Mum. He went into her room from where I overheard his goodbye message: "Okay, Mum, I'm off now. I am going to turn your radio volume up. Bye." And off he went. Fergus finds it very difficult to show his emotions. At least he has now said goodbye, with her in an intelligent state of mind. On the way to the airport we agreed that she had possibly another two weeks to live. He was sorry he had to go back to his job, as he would have liked to be here for the funeral. If Mum lived until the end of the year, he said, he would be able to take more leave to come back.

When I returned she smiled and whispered, "It's just like before."

The Last Waltz: Love, Death & Betrayal

Mum is finding it harder to speak as her tongue has become quite badly infected with a yeast or fungus. She refuses to allow the district nurses to treat it. She believes acceptance of any treatment at all would go against her absolute determination to die. This infection began a month ago on the last night she ate; we both sat down with a large packet of salt and vinegar potato crisps and finished them. She enjoyed them but later that night complained how sore her tongue was. The next morning she told me she couldn't eat any more potato crisps. As it turned out, she didn't eat anything else again. Since then her tongue has got steadily worse.

This afternoon I asked the district nurse if Mum could have a morphine drip. She said, "It is not such a straightforward request when the person is not in a hospice."

Tonight when we were talking Mum said to me, "I am going to tell you a secret." I told her that I didn't believe she had any secrets. She continued, "I will tell you where it is tomorrow." Mary interrupted this conversation with a phone call. She chatted to me and then briefly with Mum. After that I wasn't feeling in the mood for discussing Mum's secret. For Mum to tell me "where it is" is a little bizarre. Perhaps she wants to tell me where another diary is hidden.

Truffle knows things are not right and is a bit confused as to what's going on. I am so exhausted from lack of sleep I am running out of strength even to help Truffle through this crisis in her life.

I have decided to have Truffle put down when Mum dies, even though Mum wants Jo to take her. I'm sure Jo won't mind. If she takes her, Truffle will get lost in the West Coast bush and have a horrible end. Truffle is a spoilt cat who feels she is human. She will never get this attention again, and in death will be at peace like Mum.

I didn't give Mum any morphine today. I wanted to clear her system of the drug so she could think more rationally about her plan now that Fergus has gone. I think she is now incapable of taking her own life because she is too weak. I am certainly not going to assist her as I have not had a categorical instruction to do it. She said she wanted to kill herself tonight. I was not confident that she was speaking with a sound mind, and told her I would speak to her tomorrow about it. I also wanted to ask her about having Truffle put down.

Monday 23 October 2006
Day thirty-one of only water: half a cup.

Again she asks me the time, and again she wishes it were much later. Someone who has pain or fear cannot wait. She is just waiting on the edge. Waiting to die.

She is consumed by pain as her body decays. The days are long, and the nights are even longer. She is longing to die, yet afraid of the uncertainty of death.

I am so exhausted. This grief is killing me.

She asks if any doctor is going to help her. I can't think what to tell her.

Eventually I slowly whispered, "I can't believe I'm saying this, Mum, but it's never going to happen. Doctors think if they stall long enough people will die. They are more than happy to play God by keeping people alive long past their natural time, but they will never play God by easing their suffering, by helping them go a little earlier."

She sighed in resignation.

I continued, "Doctors are only doing what their profession allows them to do. It is the public and the politicians who can't find the compassion to ease that distance between dying and death. You must just wait."

I have stopped all visitors. She was pleased when I told her this. I also don't want company at this time. Mum is in such a sad state I can't bear people coming just to look at her.

It is a terrible sight. Under her bed sheets Mum has a colostomy bag on one side, and a catheter tube with a collection bag on the other. The catheter tube keeps getting blocked because of the lack of urine to flush it. Her legs cannot move at all. Her hands move a bit. Her body is little more than skin over bones. Her head is bald from the radiotherapy. Her body is covered with little sores. Her tongue has become infected. It is painful for her to talk. She is sleeping most of the time. She needs to be turned every two hours, day and night. Her body is aching with pain when

The Last Waltz: Love, Death & Betrayal

moved. In spite of this, when the morphine wears off her brain is functioning normally. Extraordinary as it seems, this state could continue for some time. The absurdity of it all is that Mum could last longer than Bobby Sands.

This is ghastly.

It is too unbelievable. Mum is literally falling to bits. The only rational thing to do is to take her to hospital or a hospice. What kind of sane person would keep their mother in a bedroom to rot to death? No one in their right mind would. Should I be roundly condemned for allowing this to happen?

This is horrific and sickening. How can this be happening?

How will I be judged for this course I am taking?

How will I be judged if I don't continue with this course of action?

To send her to hospital now, against her final wishes, would sentence me to a lifetime's damnation. I would be consumed by my own guilt.

Only I have a duty. I should not have to think about it. I made a promise to Mum to honor her Living Will. When I agreed to this, it seemed such a reasonable thing. No one questioned her decision for a second. But no one could have foreseen the sight that is before me now. No one could have imagined her skin bruising and sticking to my fingers, the smell of her rotting flesh, a tongue that is completely decayed and bedsores that make you wince at their sight.

We need help.

Things got out of control so quickly, they just snowballed. I have embarked on a path that I could never have imagined would end up in a place from which there is no return. A promise is a promise. How can the last thing I do for Mum be the breaking of a solemn promise to her? How will she feel as I carry her away from her own home to the sterile surrounds of a hospice, her devoted son cheating her at her final breath?

No, it is not an issue. It is simple. Mum has not changed her desire to die this way.

I have to honor her wish. My commitment is to the end of the line, her last breath.

The Last Waltz: Love, Death & Betrayal

Each time I turn her she still mutters, "You are such a good boy." She understands the situation I am in. We are both in this trap and are suffering together. Her words are enough to keep our connection alive. She keeps asking to die. Does she feel resentment towards me for ignoring her?

I think of all the knowledge, wisdom, and talent she cultivated in her life. Look at her now. Why do we bother with life, for it to end like this? Is life worth it just to pass the knowledge to the next unappreciative generation? How could she deserve this death? I wonder about God in all of this. I want to hate Him, but doing so makes Him exist.

Later the same day

Mum was able to chat in a soft voice tonight without the influence of morphine. She said she was going to swallow some pills to end everything. I told her that it would be difficult for her to do this since she has now got to the point where she swallows so slowly. This was a devastating blow to her. She didn't ask me to help.

I asked her if she minded if I had Truffle put down after she died. I told her that Truffle was almost certainly going to die a horrible death alone in the bush if Jo takes her, and if I have her put down she will have a peaceful one. It would be a mercy killing of an old cat. Mum didn't agree and wants Truffle to keep living with Jo.

Mum is making a bad decision. It makes much more sense to put Truffle down and let her die peacefully rather than of starvation. I wish I could ask Truffle.

Later when I was saying goodnight to Mum she whispered to me, "The morphine tablets could be crushed into a powder."

Tuesday 24 October 2006
Day thirty-two of only water: half a cup.

It was a difficult night as Mum has little strength to lift her bell and ring it. I have to be at her side most of the time now. Mum's body smells of acetone as a result of ketosis (the breakdown of the flesh to keep the organs functioning). Only

The Last Waltz: Love, Death & Betrayal

fifty percent of people can smell acetone. Fortunately I am one who can't. The district nurse said today that her skin is also starting to break down. When I turn her I have been inflicting bruises all over her body, merely from my hand pressure. Just now I left bruises on her chin from holding her face while she sipped the water. She has infections and is in pain.

I am losing my identity, unable to think. As Mum is dependent on me, so am I on her. My every moment is her life. When she is thirsty, I bring her water; when she moves, I turn her body; when she sleeps, I sleep; when she wakes, I wake; when she breathes, I breathe.

As I rearranged her pillow tonight she pleaded, "No, put it on top of my face." I told her that a pillow was no way to die. Tears ran down her face.

Mum has no morphine in her system now. I asked her clearly, "Do you really want me, your son, to be the person to give you your death wish?"

She replied, "Please, I want you to help me die." And then, "You really are a good boy." I think I have no choice but to do the unthinkable.

I am watching her sleep now.

Mum, you always said how similar I am to your father. I'm not sure if you really meant it or just wanted to believe it. This role has become a heavy one for me to bear. Now I do feel like your father, and you my dependent daughter. What would he do now? He was always there for you, yet here I am beside you, uncertain and unwilling. In your dying moments you see me for the first time hesitating to assist you. In your dying breaths you have cause to criticize me. Why must it end like this?

Wednesday 25 October 2006
Day thirty-three of only water: one cup.

Mum seemed almost unconscious this morning. She didn't want to speak or swallow water. She just lay calmly, perhaps in a different world already. I wondered if she was going soon. But like Mum, I have stopped believing it.

The Last Waltz: Love, Death & Betrayal

When the nurses came before lunch, I insisted she be given a morphine drip so she could be on a constant supply. I said that her doctor had told me she could have such a drip if she was either in unbearable pain, or having difficulties swallowing fluids. The nurses contacted her doctor, who was going to fax a script to the hospital for a nurse to come and set up a drip later today. I couldn't believe it, a morphine drip, finally. I also requested another night visit from Belinda the hospice nurse. At least Mum has got to know Belinda and is comfortable with her.

Now I am working at a table in Mum's room. Her classical music is playing in the background. I am playing her favorite Thomas Tallis CDs, which have grown on me. Occasionally I sit by her bedside and talk to her. She acknowledges my presence, but doesn't want to talk. I think she is still smarting from my telling her that she was not capable of ending her life on her own.

When the hospital phoned to confirm a nurse was coming later with the morphine drip, I knew the time had come when Mum could take an overdose in the knowledge that if excessive morphine is detected in her blood, it would be put down to the drip. She had half-heartedly referred to this as her "exit opportunity." Although it was Mum's own plan, I carefully explained to her how I would help her end her life tonight. I showed her the tablets and said that I was going to crush them into a powder she could drink once the morphine drip was in place. Her eyes lit up but she didn't speak. I asked her to nod if she understood that the drip was coming. She nodded, but there was disbelief in her eyes. She didn't believe her life would ever end. She certainly didn't believe I had the strength to help her when she knew how devoted I was to her. Perhaps she saw the uncertainty in my eyes. I still doubted my own conviction.

I wanted Mum to know that all her children were with her. I said, "Mary phones me every day. She always says she wishes she could have stayed with you." As I mentioned Mary's name Mum's eyes opened wide. I added that Mary was coming back soon. I told her that Jo also phones every day and that Fergus was back in England and would be phoning soon. She nodded in understanding.

The Last Waltz: Love, Death & Betrayal

I just gave her a hug and put my cheek next to hers. As I did this, she pushed her cheek against mine. She then opened her eyes wide and stared at me and tried to say something, but she couldn't get the words out because her tongue was so sore. I told her not to speak as there was no need to say anything more. She had already told me everything. To check that she was still understanding me I asked her to smile, and she did.

She seems strangely content about getting a morphine drip now, but oddly enough a few days ago when Doug Ogle was here and I discussed having such a drip, she didn't want one as she said it might "go wrong." I think she feared ending up in a coma for the rest of her days. That same day I had chatted with Doug when he was leaving, and I was returning from my hike. I asked him his view on helping Mum to take her own life. He told me that she had asked him several times, and he said he couldn't do it. This made me realize how serious Mum was, as Doug was a good friend with a big heart and of sound mind. He was the perfect person to help her. I also realized that since Mum had asked Doug while I was available she really wanted to protect me from being the person to help her.

I can understand Mum not wanting me to be involved in such a heart-wrenching act.

I can understand her asking Doug, the son of her best friend.

I can understand Doug refusing to help.

I can now understand my destiny.

Later the same day

About 7.30pm the nurses came and set up a morphine syringe feeder. It now seems so wrong that Mum waited so long for this. We now have the cover in place.

After they left Mum seemed more alert and asked for a glass of water. I could hardly believe it but she drank the whole lot. She then uttered her first words for the day, "I'm so parched." It dawned on me that Mum had been acting all day.

The Last Waltz: Love, Death & Betrayal

Before long Mum began moaning in pain. Initially I thought this was a consequence of the needle from the drip, but she said there was no pain where the needle was. I kept trying to find out the source of this pain. She couldn't tell me, she just said, "All over." I thought if the pain were due to some organ giving up after her long hunger strike, the source of the pain would be very obvious. I couldn't understand how it could suddenly be all over her body.

"I want to die! I've had enough!" she cried. This was followed by the most profound line that has ever crossed her lips, "Who caused all this?" She has never believed in a greater power.

Then she threw me a curve ball, "Bash me on the head!"

I told her that wouldn't kill her.

She replied, "It will help. I can't do anything. I'm finished," and continued with her moaning. I sat in horror and disbelief. The noise of my mother suffering was agony for me.

I tried to collect myself. I thought and thought. I knew the answer to the question I was posing myself. I said, "Mum, you deserve to die. You don't deserve this suffering."

"Yes," she quickly agreed. She then affirmed, "I want to die tonight. I feel dreadful. I feel pain everywhere, and I can hardly talk."

There was no doubt now. I prepared what I calculated would be a lethal drink of crushed morphine tablets.

I held it in front of her and said, "If you take this you will die." I wanted to be sure, so absolutely sure, that there was no hesitation.

She answered, "You are a wonderful son." I needed to hear it at that moment.

I said, "It is not how you planned it. It is not what I planned. This is an event that will live long after you die."

"No one will ever know."

No one will ever know, that is true, but I will. Her destiny is not in her hands as she planned it, but in mine.

I held the glass to her lips and gently poured the liquid into her mouth. She had no difficulty in swallowing her last glass. She looked at me with a gentle smile.

I looked at her, "Has the time come for our last waltz?"

The Last Waltz: Love, Death & Betrayal

"On the other side," she mumbled.

I said, "But you don't believe in the other side."

She paused and said, "But you do," and closed her eyes.

Mum is full of wisdom and has never sinned. I think she will be at a very high level on the other side, maybe approaching Nirvana. Perhaps this dreadful death is her final test.

I hugged her. As I went to rinse out the glass I thought how devastated she would be if once again, after all this, and after all we had just been through, she were to wake up in the morning yet again... But surely this time she wouldn't? Surely? Though I could just imagine her saying, "I told you I am immortal."

Mum stopped speaking for some time as I held her but sometimes gently moaned.

She was receiving a minimal dose of morphine from the drip. I thought she should get extra from the night nurse, who was coming later. This extra dose would explain the high dose of morphine in her blood, and move any suspicion away from me.

I phoned Belinda and explained that Mum was in great pain (she groaned loudly in the background for effect) and told her that she would need to give her extra morphine. Belinda was quite in agreement with this as she could hear Mum, but she said she would have to get a doctor's permission.

About an hour later Belinda arrived and entered the house through the balcony door. I was sitting on the side of Mum's bed. As soon as Mum saw Belinda she looked aghast and called out, "Go, Go!" I was taken aback by this reaction as Mum had really liked Belinda when she stayed the previous week.

I realized that Mum saw Belinda as another person trying to keep her alive. I turned to Mum and said, "It's okay, Mum, Belinda won't keep you alive."

Mum's facial expression immediately softened and she smiled and mumbled, "Thank God."

Belinda said there was a problem, as she could not administer extra morphine. She had been unable to get hold of a doctor to get permission to do so.

The Last Waltz: Love, Death & Betrayal

Mum said nothing. I think the evening's events were overwhelming.

I asked Belinda to leave us alone for a while. I then whispered into Mum's ear, "Mum, you have carried off tonight with aplomb."

She replied with barely audible words, "Yes, I am now dying in style." Again she had that enchanting smile, indicating that the whole evening had been cleverly managed on her part, to seek the escape from this life that she so desperately wanted.

I kept reassuring Mum that her death must be near, although I think she was still a little skeptical. I then thought of words to make her happy. "Mum, your hair is growing back. It's starting to look very nice again."

She heard me and her eyes sparkled, as she obviously loved to hear this. I was deluding myself because if it were growing back it would only be very short stubble. What I meant was that she was looking beautiful, as she was so willingly and painlessly moving towards her death. Her hair, her smile, everything was beautiful as she lay there so relaxed and perhaps a little smug, perhaps thinking that she had finally won by outsmarting the people who were intent on keeping her alive.

Mum kept trying to say something to me, but she couldn't get the words out clearly. She tried and tried. I told her not to say anything now, and that we had said our goodbyes many times over. She understood me. I said to her, "Just smile at me if you understand everything that is going on." She smiled. There was no doubt she was happy.

Belinda returned and described to me the normal pattern of events as a body approaches death. Belinda felt Mum's toes and commented on the coldness of them, and how this was sometimes an indication of approaching death. She said that the cold would spread up her body. I was relieved at hearing this, although it crossed my mind that Mum always had cold toes. I kept talking to Mum to reassure her that this really was the end.

At midnight I thought that Mum was almost where she wanted to be. I decided to phone Mary so she could say goodbye. I felt it was the right thing to do because Mum had said that Mary wanted to be there at the very end.

I phoned her in Melbourne, about four hours behind us, and by an extraordinary coincidence she was having a candlelight wake for Mum with her youngest daughter. Neither of us could believe this. Mary asked me to put the phone to Mum's ear, which I did. She then gave her farewell speech, saying how wonderful she was, and how she would miss her. She then said, "Say something, Mum, just so I know that you are listening and understand." Mum was nodding her head and was able to mumble down the phone, which thrilled Mary. Mum was also very moved to hear Mary speaking to her. I told her I would call her back as soon as Mum had gone.

Mum continued trying to speak but the words were totally incomprehensible. I said, "I'm sorry, Mum, I can't understand you." I felt terrible as I'd always been the one who'd been able to understand her over the past few weeks. I could translate when her voice was soft and fading and her visitors didn't understand her. Now, at the time when she was uttering her last words, I was unable to hear. I thought of nodding and agreeing with her and pretending I could hear, but this seemed so dishonest when we were at this moment of truth. The time for deception was over. Instead I said, "Mum, you and I have said everything we need to say to each other. You don't need to say anything. Just sleep." She seemed to understand.

Another hour went by and Mum was still wide-awake. Belinda was wondering why she hadn't gone to sleep, and asked if I had given her Mogadon. I told her I hadn't. It hadn't crossed my mind. She said that this was the reason Mum wasn't sleeping. Then she said she didn't think Mum was near death tonight. This was a frightening thought.

I realized that Belinda's belief that Mum was near death had not come from any medical assessment but from feeding off my certainty that I had given her enough morphine to end her life. Perhaps I was wrong. I was now in a state of panic and again asked Belinda to inject Mum with extra morphine. She refused, saying that she was not allowed to.

The Last Waltz: Love, Death & Betrayal

Belinda was going to do nothing to help. She assessed Mum and said that she was certain she was not going to die as the coolness in her toes had not spread and her breathing had stayed constant.

I phoned Mary to tell her this development, and she said "I'm sick of this." She had already booked her ticket to New Zealand since our previous call, and was coming to Dunedin tomorrow.

It must have been about 1am when I started dozing off to sleep next to Mum. Mum was breathing heavily, but sleeping. I allowed myself to sleep, too, until Belinda shook me awake. She said, "Your mother is dead." I wrapped my arms around Mum and squeezed her and said, "You are free, Mum! Thank God, you are free!"

The Last Waltz: Love, Death & Betrayal

PART THREE

Betrayal

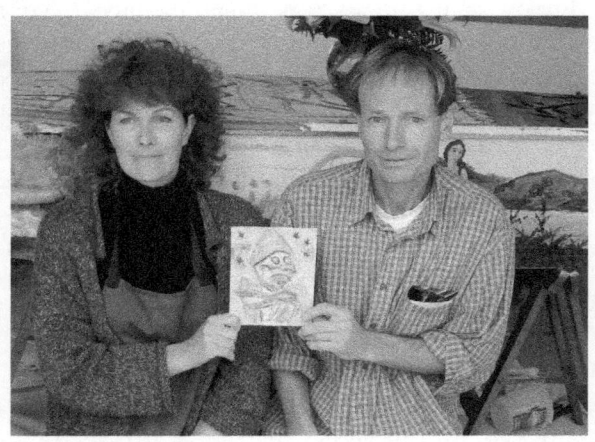

Every day confirms my opinion on the superiority of a vicious life - and if Virtue is not its own reward I don't know any other stipend annexed to it.

Lord Byron

The Last Waltz: Love, Death & Betrayal

FOUR YEARS LATER

Hotel Singapore: September 2010

These stop-offs at Hotel Singapore are usually a welcome bit of time out from the real world, but this time I can't avoid the media story about the big 7.4 earthquake in Christchurch, New Zealand. Miraculously, no one was killed, but it seems there was huge damage. I've tried Skyping Jo, but there's no reply. I'll try again once I get to the conference in Sydney tomorrow.

I hadn't planned to go to New Zealand – but perhaps I should.

Australia: Next day

"I'm glad you're okay, but I'm going to come to Christchurch after the conference. I'm so close – you're only across the ditch."

"I'd love to see you, but it's not necessary."

"I'm insisting. I'll be there."

"Aren't you worried about the police investigating that you helped Mum to die?"

"Nope. They want my case to disappear and be forgotten. Nothing will happen."

"You're probably right. Let me know when you're arriving and I'll try to meet you. It might be difficult, as a lot of the inner-city roads are closed because of damage."

Jo's concerns about the police investigating Mum's death are understandable. I still can't get over that dreadful one line email from Mary:

"Sean, I'm reporting you to the police for murdering our mother."

She was so desperate to stop the publication of my diary (which I published as a book), that there was no telling what she might do. The problem for Mary was that I described her as I perceived her. I was writing my diary, after all. I was careful not to be unkind, but it was difficult not to describe things as they really were. I thought everything was fine once her lawyers dropped the two court injunctions, after I made her so squeaky clean she was like an angel. However, when a copy of the book's manuscript mysteriously found its way to the offices of the *New Zealand Herald*, it was hard not to suspect Mary. I guess the police were obliged to carry out a token investigation once the newspaper made a meal out of it. I think the fact that I didn't describe in the published book that I actually assisted Mum to die should be enough to placate the police. But the newspaper had the original manuscript… the smoking gun. I heard from some of the people mentioned in the book that the police interviewed them, but they all said that the detectives always implied they were doing what they were told and didn't want to be investigating such an act of compassion.

Christchurch, New Zealand: Next week

Coming through Christchurch airport, I was pulled from the queue and told to wait. After half an hour, they told me I had an unpaid traffic fine and had to pay it immediately or I would be arrested. I asked for more details, and it emerged that there were two unpaid fines from five years ago! Don't they have anything better to do? One was for speeding in Oamaru, and the other for Mum not wearing a seat belt while she was my passenger. I said I'd pay for the speeding ticket, but not the seat belt one, because of the circumstances at the time.

"You're giving us no choice but to arrest you."

"Be my guest, but I'm not paying it on principle."

The officer squirmed. "The local cells are quake-damaged, with water everywhere. You'll be uncomfortable."

"Comfort isn't the issue."

The two cops looked at each other, went into a back room, and returned ten minutes later. "Head office in Wellington says you can go for now, but must pay before you leave the country or you'll be arrested then."

I didn't argue. I'd rather return to fight another day.

The Last Waltz: Love, Death & Betrayal

I'm at Jo's now and have already experienced several aftershocks. At one point I was speaking by phone to a friend on the other side of Christchurch and he said, "Did you feel that?"

"No." I replied, then a few seconds later the ground shook under the house.

It's quite unsettling, but at the same time, I'm enjoying the novelty. It's easy to be blasé when I didn't experience the big one.

I'm renting a car tomorrow and heading to Dunedin.

Monday 20 September 2010

Good God! The police want to question me about Mum's death. I don't believe it. I hope it's just a formality so that they can tell the public there's insufficient evidence and the investigation is finished. When I was at Ian's yesterday, they phoned and asked if he knew where I was, and loyal Ian said I was in the country "somewhere" but he had no idea where. At that moment, Sandra called out from the kitchen, "Do you want a cup of tea, Sean?"

Today Jo phoned to say the police had contacted her to ask me to turn myself in for questioning at the Dunedin police station. She phoned again tonight to say they had arrived unannounced at her door in Christchurch, looking for me. When they said they had driven up from Dunedin, she told them I was in Dunedin! They asked if they could take a statement from her and were really pissed off when she said she was too busy as she had an exam tomorrow.

I'm staying in a motel in Dunedin so they can't find me. I think I'd better leave the country. In fact, no "thinking" about it, I definitely will. I'll phone Singapore Airlines tomorrow. This will probably be doing the police a big favor, since I'm sure they don't really want to investigate the case. It'll be a surprise for Ian when I phone him from the international departures lounge.

The Last Waltz: Love, Death & Betrayal

Tuesday 21 September 2010

They thumped at my motel room door while I was still asleep. There were two police detectives outside when I opened up.

"Are you Sean Davison?"

"Yes."

"We would like to ask you questions concerning a manuscript which describes the death of your mother."

My heart raced as I told myself to keep calm. I remembered the advice Chris Catley's lawyer had given me and knew not to say anything that could be used against me. I had his one line ready for this eventuality.

"The manuscript is fantasy, my book is what happened." I lied. I wanted to make them think they were wasting their time and give up. Phew, I had really said it. "I've arranged Skype calls this morning to my university in South Africa, so can I pop down at lunchtime?" I continued, following Jo's delaying tactics.

"Umm, I suppose," one mumbled, taken aback by my confidence. "We'll expect you at twelve, then."

This gave me time to phone Roger Laybourn, a lawyer I had contacted when the newspaper first ran the story. I told him what had happened.

"Say nothing," he said immediately. "I need my powder dry if I'm going to defend you."

Later the same day

I went meticulously through every folder on my laptop and deleted everything related to my book. Any paperwork I put into a plastic bag and threw into a street bin on my way to the police station.

At the station I was led into an interview room by two detectives. Detective Verry sat with me at a small table with some electronic recording devices. Detective Nichols sat alone, away from the table.

"Sean, I would like to ask you some questions concerning the death of your mother on October 25th 2006," said Detective Verry.

The Last Waltz: Love, Death & Betrayal

"Am I under arrest?"

"No you're not, and you're under no obligation to answer the questions," he said.

"It's okay, I'm willing to answer." I wanted to appear co-operative, but was confident I knew where to the draw the line.

He turned on the video camera and placed a manuscript with a police cover in front of me.

"Did you write this?" he asked.

"No, I didn't," I said. Why should I admit to something with a police cover? It had no resemblance to my manuscript. Okay, perhaps I wasn't being particularly co-operative.

"Please pick it up and look inside." He was irritated.

I picked it up and turned the cover. What a shock! This was not just the original manuscript, but the copy with a photo of Mum's self-portrait on the front cover. This was Mary's copy. I reeled inwardly and tried to suppress a gasp.

How did they have this? Had they interviewed Mary and confiscated it? I'm sure they wanted to shock me into thinking she gave it to them – but she wouldn't do that.

"Can you confirm that you wrote this manuscript?" he persisted. I knew this was crucial information for them. They had to have confirmation from me. But Roger wanted his powder dry.

"I'm sorry, I've been advised by my Hamilton lawyer not to answer that question," I said gamely, and could sense the detectives' disappointment at my invoking my right to remain silent. Detective Verry asked me to hand over both of my passports and I agreed, though I couldn't see why it was necessary, as they could always arrest me at the airport if I tried to leave. They followed me back to the motel to collect them.

This has not been a good day in my life. I have lied to the police. I just panicked. I didn't think it would come to this. No w, for the first time, I've denied my manuscript – denied my life? I have lied to myself. I feel I've denied my own mother.

The Last Waltz: Love, Death & Betrayal

Friday 24 September 2010

"You are under arrest ..."
Oh God, no, this can't be happening.

"And charged with the attempted murder."
Murder! What the hell are they talking about?

"of Patricia Elizabeth Davison."
Patricia Davison – that's Mum. I didn't murder Mum!

"You have the right to remain silent."
For Christ's sake! This is a dream. Wake up!

"Anything you say can and will be used in evidence against you."

Raine and the kids. What will they do? I'm stuck here.

"If you wish to consult a lawyer..."

They can't cope without me. Oh Christ! I must phone Roger, he'll tell me what to do. Oh hell, I have a memory stick in my pocket with copies of the manuscript on it. It'll be a disaster if the police get hold of it. Damn it, arrested with the evidence smoking in my pocket!

We sat in silence for some minutes while arrangements were being made. I was in shock, my mind was everywhere. I knew I should bite my tongue, but I piped up anyway.

"One day you'll be waiting for your death. I hope it's an easy and dignified one, but perhaps it won't be. When that time comes, I want you to think of this moment." They looked uncomfortable.

Eventually the detectives left the room while I spoke on the phone to my lawyer.

"I need my powder dry," Roger said again. "Don't say a word. Every word you say will weaken my hand."

"Can I speak to you now, or are they listening somewhere?" I asked. "They could be listening, but they

The Last Waltz: Love, Death & Betrayal

can't use it as evidence. This is referred to as lawyer-client confidentiality. We'll talk later."

While speaking to Roger, I discreetly slipped the memory stick into my shoe, disguising the act by scratching my ankle in case they were watching through one-way glass. I had to get it out of my pocket in case I was searched. Detective Verry returned and led me to the holding cells. I felt he was a good man, but I knew I mustn't let my guard down – that they'd want to lull me into a false sense of security so I'd say things I shouldn't.

"You are going to a bail hearing once you've been processed."

Processed? Bail hearing? What's happening?

"You will be searched and you have to hand over your shoes."

My shoes! The memory stick! Damn. He must have seen me. If they find it in my shoe, it's obvious I've got something to hide. Curse that manuscript! And now I have it in my damn shoe?

My mind was all over the place. It must have been one-way glass. But that means my feeling about Detective Verry was correct. He is a good man and he's giving me a chance to avoid embarrassment when I take off my shoes. Where can I put it? Can I drop it somewhere around the station as we walk, in a pot plant, behind a fire extinguisher? Shall I ask to go to the toilet and flush it? Hide it in the tiny pocket at the top of my jeans? Swallow it? Good God! As we waited in the passage for the door to the security cells to be unlocked, I tried wiggling the memory stick to the outside rim of my shoe so I could grab it in one swoop without fiddling with my shoe.

I wasn't discreet enough, because Detective Verry looked at me, and I believe he knew. Then, luckily, he looked away, which gave me a chance. Maybe he felt I had enough problems. In the processing room I had to empty my pockets into a plastic bag, and no one noticed, while they were focusing on my jacket, that when I reached down to pull my shoe off, the memory stick popped into my hand, then magically appeared from my jacket pocket and went straight into their plastic bag. Phew, that was lucky. They've got the evidence now, but better this way than them catching me hiding it. To think I was prepared to swallow it!.

I asked Detective Verry if I could send some text messages. He gave an uncertain nod, as if to give the impression of agreeing reluctantly as a token favor, but I seized the opportunity to delete all messages from my phone, and I also deleted the lists of phone numbers dialed and received. As I did this it rang, so I quickly answered before Detective Verry could intervene.

"I've got ten bucks on the Warriors!" came Ian's voice.

"I'm in jail, Ian, I've been arrested."

"Good one. I'm not falling for that. I'm no longer an 'Ernie'."

I quickly cut the call and gave the phone to the disapproving detective, expressing my gratitude and telling him I had sent a message to my partner in South Africa. Detective Verry put the cell phone and memory stick in a separate plastic bag, saying, "I'll take care of these and get them back to you quickly." That was a relief.

"What is this?" he asked, looking at the memory stick as he wrote down a list of my possessions. I wondered where he'd been the last fifteen years. Perhaps he'll give these back after my bail hearing without investigating them further.

The "processing" continued. It was just like the movies, right down to the mug shot in front of a wall holding a number card, and a swab from the inside of my cheek for DNA profiling. I was physically searched and asked to remove my belt, and my shoes were returned without the laces. Apparently this is a normal procedure to prevent suicides – suicide by shoelace?

"Come this way, Sean, we're driving you to court now," said the middle-aged officer respectfully. "This way. Just take a seat in there for a wee while," and he pointed to a metal cage in the back of the police van. The door closed and the key turned.

I was locked in the back of a police van. I could never have imagined this happening. The van had another sealed cage behind me, and I heard him much less politely put two other guys in there. Then the van drove to the nearby court, which seemed to be underground.

The Last Waltz: Love, Death & Betrayal

"Come this way, Sean. You have to wait in a holding cell until you're called to the court."

Good God, a holding cell.

I was put in a cell with the two thugs that had also been in the police van. They seemed very rough, covered in tattoos and speaking in expletives. My initial reaction was to fear for my safety, as they could see that I wasn't like them and might take a dislike to me. Though I had no idea what they were in here for, it seemed that if they were at rock bottom and had nothing to lose, they might do anything. I sat on the concrete bench, leaning over and staring at my shoes. Damn that memory stick.

"Hey, mate, how'd they get to write on these walls?" said one of my cellmates. "Everyone brought here is stripped of all their shit, so how come these walls are covered in all them words?"

It was a good point. The walls were covered in abusive graffiti.

We introduced ourselves. They were decent guys, nothing like their external images. One of them was then taken away to the court. The other told me he'd been arrested for not reporting for bail – that he had to sign in each week, had just lost track of the days, and was now back in court. He was out on bail for approaching his ex-wife, who had a restraining order against him. He gave a detailed description of how the wife had set him up and what a bitch she was. It sounded convincing to me.

I told him about the charge against me. I said I was in shock because I wouldn't be able to go back home to South Africa, since they had my passports.

"South Africa, I've been there," he said. "I worked on a fishing boat for a couple of years and I had a trip to Mauritius, Madagascar and South Africa." I believed him since his geographical knowledge was so good.

"A fishing boat," I pondered aloud. "That's the only way I can get back to my family now."

"That can be arranged," he said with a wink.

The Last Waltz: Love, Death & Betrayal

At that moment the policeman came to the door to fetch him. Suddenly, I realized, I may need this man.

"What's your name?" I quickly asked as he was led out the door.

"Kris Martin," he told me, adding that he lived in Mosgiel. "My number's in the phone book." He knew my intention.

A fishing boat? Yes, I may have to consider that option. I had no pen but had to make sure I wouldn't forget his name. Under my present stress I could lose it easily. I focused my mind – I mustn't forget his name. I wish I could scratch it on the wall. How did they write that graffiti?

Next it was my turn, and the detective led me to the court, from the dim holding cell, through a cold grey passageway, then suddenly into the daunting courtroom filled with people, the most intimidating high on the front bench in full regalia. The detective indicated for me to step up into the witness stand. Dazed and shocked, I struggled to understand his instruction.

"Mr. Davison, you are charged with the attempted murder of Patricia Elizabeth Davison," the woman judge called out. "Do you have legal counsel in the court?"

"I'm not sure," I meekly replied, not knowing if this comes automatically as part of the package. "I don't think so."

"Can someone tell me if this man has legal representation here?" she demanded.

"No, ma'am," said an officer. "He was only arrested this afternoon, but the police are not opposing his bail."

"What's that?" the judge exclaimed. "The police don't oppose bail? This is a charge of attempted murder. I oppose bail!"

What the hell is going on here?

"Ma'am, this is a historical case from 2006. We don't oppose bail," the officer repeated.

"But I do!" the judge roared again.

My heart sank. Am I going to be in the Dunedin prison for the weekend – and for who knows how long after that?

How can I get the word out? Roger? I was motionless, in shock.

"Can anyone give me a summary of this case?" the judge asked.

"No, ma'am," said the detective. "Mr. Davison was only arrested this afternoon and I don't have a charge sheet ready."

"This is not good enough. The defendant has no representation, and no one can give me a summary of the case."

Oh God, I've got to do something – quickly.

"Excuse me, ma'am," I spoke up timidly. "I'm sorry to interrupt, but could I give you a little summary, please?"

"You certainly cannot," the judge roared at me, presumably horrified that a defendant was interrupting her. She then stared at me for some moments; perhaps I didn't look like the run-of-the-mill matricide type, for she continued with a twinkle in her eye: "We shall see. Perhaps I will ask you for a wee summary when you come back."

Thank heavens. That worked out okay. Maybe she has some compassion.

I was led from the court to another holding cell, so that my case could be discussed. The court duty lawyer was then quickly advised of my details and presented them to the judge in my absence, but it was about twenty or thirty minutes before I was led back to hear her decision. I was feeling more confident, for surely she would have now learnt about my book and be more sympathetic.

"You are charged with a very serious crime, the attempted murder of your mother, Patricia Elizabeth Davison, on 25 October 2006. A crime such as this does not make it easy for me to grant you bail." My heart sank. "I also have to take into consideration whether you are likely to repeat the offence if I grant you bail. However, I don't think you are likely to commit euthanasia again," and she again looked at me with a naughty smile. "I grant you bail until Tuesday morning, nine am."

The Last Waltz: Love, Death & Betrayal

What a relief. But, what a cheek to suggest I wouldn't commit euthanasia *again*: she is already finding me guilty. But at least she freed me from the cells for the weekend.

The court duty lawyer came to chat to me after the hearing. He was very smooth as he gave me his card.

"You can contact me any time, day or night," he said. "Your book was a fine piece of fiction, wasn't it?" He gave me a wink.

"Fiction?" I meekly asked, wondering how he'd come up with that idea. "Oh yes, I suppose so."

"I'm happy to represent you in the trial."

"Okay. Thanks." I felt relief to know I had a friendly lawyer in Dunedin in case Roger didn't come through. Meanwhile, I have to go back to court on Tuesday to have my bail conditions reviewed. Detective Verry led me back to my car, which was now in the police garage under the station. He apologized for not having been able to bring a sandwich to my cell. I believe he tried.

"This is crazy, to be arrested for helping my mother as I did," I said to him, unsure of how open I should be.

"Sorry, Sean, but police are not allowed to have an opinion."

Hmmm ... He's on my side.

Back at my motel

I have to stay at this motel.

They executed a search warrant while I was in court, and everything has been pulled out. They've confiscated my electronic stuff, including my laptop, both cell phones, camera and memory sticks, and all of my paperwork. My room feels contaminated, assaulted, raped.

I've spoken to the motel owners in an attempt to calm them down, since having cops searching their units can't be good for business – and, even worse, they now have an accused murderer in residence. I told them about my mother, my book, my arrest – and they couldn't get enough of it, saying I could have the room for half price, which is a relief, since I have to stay here till my next hearing. If they'd forced me out I would've had to go to the police cells,

The Last Waltz: Love, Death & Betrayal

because only the court can decide my address – and it doesn't sit again until next week.

This is going to be a bumpy ride. What to do now? They're still asleep in Cape Town. I'll phone Raine later. Yep, a bumpy ride.

Jesus! What about my job?

My air tickets? I'll miss my booked flight. What date do I change them to? Next year? Longer?

And the rental car. How do I get that back to Christchurch? It'll cost a packet.

Lawyers too, for that matter. I hate to think about that. If this goes to trial, I could be bankrupted for life. I'm not working in South African rands now; this is all in New Zealand dollars, one of the world's stronger currencies.

Oh God, how can I tell Chris Catley? She's my publisher. She'll feel terrible for publishing the book. But it wasn't the book, it was the manuscript that caused this mess, and that's not her fault. I hope she'll be okay. Damn the manuscript! How on earth did it find its way out there?

I have name suppression for the time being, meaning that the media can't report who appeared in court for the attempted murder of their mother. Maybe by the time this suppression is lifted next week, the whole thing will have blown away and they'll have dropped the charges. Yes, if that could only happen! This is such nonsense.

During the night

Damn it, I can't sleep. I may as well just stay up all night.

I've spoken to Raine. That's one off my list. She kept pretty cool, and at least she's got her parents, Ouma and Oupa there, to help with our boys.

I told her my plan is to say the manuscript is fiction, so she's undertaken to destroy all of my documents at the house, just in case they have a way of getting a search warrant in South Africa. Of course it's unlikely, but I can't take a chance, as things have become serious.

Raine's main concern is our financial situation, if things go badly, if this goes to court. A court case won't come cheap, and she's worried I may lose my job. I've still got to get my mind around my job, but perhaps if I just keep quiet, and if things go well, the university will never know.

I can't speak to anyone without my laptop to Skype from, and it's too late for anyone to call me back, since the call will have to go through the motel reception. Everything's a mess.

Later the same night

Oh bugger, bugger, bugger. How did they get Mary's manuscript? She hasn't told anyone she was interviewed by the police.

Saturday 25 September 2010

I'm moving to Ian's brother's place today. John is a thoroughly decent guy who I've known as long as Ian. In fact, he's stored a trunk load of my belongings for the past twenty-two years, waiting for me to collect them. Unlike Ian, he doesn't have a house full of kids. In fact, he lives alone with his fifteen-year-old cat, Putter. He's not charging me anything, which I appreciate.

Living on South African rands and buying in New Zealand dollars is really going to strain the budget.

Later the same day

I've just had a long hike up to the top of Mount Cargill. I'm feeling a mixture of euphoria and depression. The euphoria is from the hope that my fiction plan will lead to the charges being dropped and this will get me back to Cape Town. The depression is because I feel helpless, stuck here, unable to save myself. Day and night my mind is focused on what I wrote in my manuscript and working out alternative fictitious meanings. Every night I toss and turn, thinking of new angles, new traps, new riddles – and let's be honest – new lies. How on earth did I find myself in this situation, where I'm planning the best strategy to lie to a court of law?

The Last Waltz: Love, Death & Betrayal

It doesn't feel good, but I'm feeling so desperate. I'm not a murderer... nor am I a liar.

Later the same night

"Sorry Sean, your fiction plan is no good," Ian just told me on the phone. "Deleting all of the manuscript drafts from your laptop won't work because they can get into the hard drive and access all deleted material. You see, last year I did this teacher workshop about tracking pedophiles by analyzing their computer hard drives, and I've just dug out my notes."

"No. Surely when you delete stuff and empty your trash it's gone? I've deleted masses of stuff over the years. It can't all still be there."

"It will take them a while, but it is all stored somewhere. They just do a search for key words and find what they need. I've heard of this in other cases."

"I hope you're wrong. But I can still say it's fiction."

"Is there anything else incriminating, apart from the manuscript?"

"Well, yes, there's correspondence with Chris Catley. That was also deleted – but you say it's still there."

"Then you need to have stories to cover everything, otherwise you're going to be tripping all over yourself."

"The main thing is that they don't have me saying first-hand that I did it. Everything they find will be circumstantial evidence."

"And since they searched your motel room they probably bugged your phone."

"What! They can't do that!"

"Oh yes they can, and there have been a number of recent cases where the police have gone over the top in their electronic surveillance. You had better be more careful."

I was flabbergasted. "If this motel phone is bugged I'm history. I've had several conversations with you and Raine, where I've outlined my fiction strategy."

"They're probably listening now."

"I may as well make a full confession. I'm going to fry."

The Last Waltz: Love, Death & Betrayal

This could change everything. I have to find out if my phone's bugged so I can plan ahead. I can't just wait and find out when I'm in the dock. Also, I need a local Dunedin lawyer. It won't work with Roger up there. I need someone I can see any time I need to. I'm going to phone Len Andersen tomorrow, as he's been recommended. There have been several calls from lawyers offering their services, but I think they just want a high-profile case to advance their careers, which doesn't engender much confidence.

Mind you, if they're desperate for my case, perhaps they'll do it cheaply. I've had estimates ranging from R200 000 to R400 000 for this type of criminal trial.

Later the same day

I'm impressed by Len Andersen, especially because of his reluctance to meet me today, even though he'd heard about my case. He actually wanted to wait until Monday, despite my bail hearing being on Tuesday, thereby running the risk of me finding another lawyer in the meantime. But how could I wait?

Anyway, Len must have detected my anxiety because he agreed to meet me outside his office at one pm. If he hadn't, I would have definitely taken the next lawyer on my list. I'm too anxious to wait.

I liked Len's relaxed, unpretentious demeanor. Sure, he was in jeans and T-shirt because it's a Saturday afternoon, but he seemed a man with nothing to prove.

We went to his office, where I told him the whole story. Well, it is a story – it's certainly not the truth – and I'm sticking to it. I told him that the manuscript was fiction and I just wanted to sensationalize it to make it sell better, and that my book was the true story. I said if the police had only asked me right at the start, they could have avoided all of this. I spoke without hesitation. I was so damn convincing I believed myself. He said he would like to take the case. He couldn't give a price, since it was dependent on many factors. I kept pushing him for an indication, but he wasn't even prepared to give a ballpark figure.

The Last Waltz: Love, Death & Betrayal

I like Len. He seems like a good lateral thinker – important in this case, which will be full of riddles as the prosecution and defense tussle over whether lines in my manuscript are fact or fiction. I didn't tell Len what they might find deleted on my laptop, and what they'll have heard if they bugged my motel phone. Lawyers are used to surprises.

Anyway, it's a relief to have decided on a lawyer, though I find myself wondering if I shouldn't have stuck with Roger, who's had so much experience in criminal cases.

Later the same night

Damn, I need sleep. My mind starts spinning at this time of the night.

I've got to keep calm. I've got to believe everything will be okay. I've got to stick to my script.

The jury will have to see some doubt and let me go. But how long will I be here? That's the hard part.

Sunday 26 September 2010

Today I needed advice from someone I trust, and I would trust Jindra Tichy with my life, as I would Ian. She was my philosophy lecturer at Otago University and is now a dear friend. I don't get to see her every time I'm back in New Zealand, because she spends half the year with relatives in the Czech Republic. We tend to see the world through the same eyes, but she can be very critical of me.

"You're a fool, Sean," Jindra said.

I asked why.

"Everything you do. You've asked Len to be your lawyer and now you have doubts and might ask someone else. Why didn't you come and talk to me before you told Len he could do it?"

"I don't have time to consult you on every decision."

"Then you are fool."

Her daughter piped up that she must stop calling me that. I agreed. I'm feeling enough stress without Jindra's abuse.

The Last Waltz: Love, Death & Betrayal

"I do have doubts about whether I chose the right lawyer in Len," I said. "But these doubts are mainly because I phoned Roger this morning and he sowed some seeds of doubt."

"Then you must live with your foolish mistakes. You can't blame anyone else."

"I don't."

Later the same day

The last time I spoke to Roger, he kept insisting that he was the country's best lawyer at working juries, that he wanted the case because it was so interesting, that he didn't need money, and that he just wanted the satisfaction of the challenge. I also kept pushing him for an indication of how much it might cost, and he too kept dodging the question. His line was that it didn't matter because he had ways of helping me raise the funds.

When I told Roger that I had given the case to Len Andersen, he replied that he wanted to fly down and see me on Monday, so he could convince me that he was the lawyer I needed. He said that he would pay for his flight, even if I didn't want him.

This has made it so confusing. Roger's very persuasive, but I've never met him. How do I know he's not just a smarmy lawyer shark? How can I be sure it's possible for him to raise funds to help me pay his fee. How can he be sure? It was kind of him not to charge me when I was first arrested, and for all the advice that followed, but if I formally appoint him as my trial lawyer, the meter starts ticking.

Choosing a lawyer or a doctor... It's all a game of chance, and you don't really know what you're getting, until it's too late.

Monday 27 September 2010

I've made the decision to stick with Len. Roger was quite magnanimous when I phoned him this morning to thank him for his assistance. He said if I changed my mind he would be there for me – and added that it was quite common to get a more junior lawyer to handle a case until it was committed to trial, and then change to the best lawyer. I won't mention this to Len!

This afternoon I had a scheduled meeting with Len to go through the case in more detail. I am getting more and more confident in my lies. I've gone through all of the possible traps the prosecutor can pull on me, and worked out how I can avoid them with my fiction story. I'm feeling optimistic, but it still seems wrong to be denying and lying.

I asked Len if I could be associated with the Voluntary Euthanasia Society. He said it was okay, since I'd stated my desire for a law change publicly during my book launch last year. Besides, he said, this all came after my mother's death and is not relevant to how she died.

Len then pulled a surprise.

"You know, Sean, if you're found guilty of attempted murder, you will lose your mother's inheritance."

Later the same night

"I have a cunning plan," Ian said after I told him I would lose my inheritance if I lost the case. "Place all your money on one bet to double your money: if you lose, you have no inheritance to give up; if you win, you give them the inheritance, keep your winnings, and you lose nothing. If you're interested, I've got some inside information on a horse racing tomorrow that can't lose."

Tuesday 28 September 2010

It was my bail hearing in court today. I'm glad Jindra turned up as support. I had no idea it would be so difficult and thought I could do it alone – but that would have been terrible. Not that I had to do anything. I just sat in the public gallery while the charge was read, then Len made a request for my bail conditions to be changed, which the judge approved. I am to report each Wednesday to the Dunedin police and reside at an address agreed to by the court (Peter Hinds's place). To avoid the media stalking me, they didn't want my address to be public knowledge. Straightforward, but still it was stressful being there.

Jindra sat next to me. "You're a fool, Sean," she began again. "You're a fool and it's part of your education to know that." I didn't want to be educated this time, so I let it rest.

Later the same night

Radio New Zealand News: *In the Dunedin District Court today Sean Davison appeared on the charge of the attempted murder of his mother Patricia Davison on October 25th 2006.*

I was preparing dinner as this came over the radio, and I froze. My name on the radio associated with murder. This is the national news, the whole country knows now. What will people think? I didn't realize that my name suppression had been lifted in the court this morning.

Thank God I'm leaving Dunedin tomorrow. This place feels like hell. The police have allowed me to drive to Christchurch to get the rental car back. Its bill is mounting and I can't delay any longer. It'll be good to catch up with Jo.

Christchurch: Thursday 30 September 2010

I spent most of the day with Jo, who's not just a good sister but a good friend. How comforting to know there are some people in the world who will stand by you no matter what happens.

It was a warm, cheerful day. The locals had brushed off the trauma of the earthquake and the several aftershocks we experienced were something of a joke. We would try guessing how big they were and then tune into the news to find out. The biggest today, when we nearly lost our coffee at the Starbucks in Cathedral Square, was 4.8 on the Richter scale.

Jo says the media have been hounding her since they couldn't find me, with journalists and cameramen staking out her house. A *New Zealand Herald* reporter has phoned many times, asking for me. She keeps brushing them off, which really irritates them. This morning one phoned and said: "How does it feel to have a brother who is a murderer?"

Jo is staying at Drew's place in Lyttelton, until they marry and leave for China at the end of the year. I'm staying alone at Jo's home in central Christchurch, a charming little upstairs-downstairs house with a small, lush, back garden. It also tends to shake quite vigorously during aftershocks. I'm surprised it survived the big quake. There have been three after-shocks while I'm writing this... I confess I'm feeling a little uneasy going to sleep...

Later, same night

God almighty! That was a helluva shock. Ian just phoned.
"They've got me Sean! The police have got me!" he bellowed down the phone.
"What do you mean? Are you under arrest?"
"I was so scared. I didn't know what to do... I told them everything."
"Calm down Ian. I don't understand? What happened?"
"They came to the house. Three of them. They said if I didn't start talking I was an accomplice... that I could go to jail... I had to think of my kids... they said they could seize my computer, with all your emails..."
"What did you tell them?"
"Everything..."

Sunday 3 October 2010

I took the bus back to Dunedin today. Six hours of staring out the window, deep in thought. I felt totally demoralized. My life seemed to be passing before my eyes.

When I got to Ian's, his wife met me at the gate.

"He's really upset. He's calling himself your Judas," she said.

I found Ian inside the house looking miserable.

The Last Waltz: Love, Death & Betrayal

"I just don't get it, Ian. We spent hours planning my fictitious defense, and then you hand the police everything on a plate."

"I'm sorry, I panicked," he mumbled. "But don't worry, I've been thinking and I have a plan…"

"It's too late. The damage is done."

"Look, I'm nearly fifty and I don't care what people think of me. I can take the stand and say I lied in my statement. I really would do that for you. I just panicked yesterday… I'll make it right."

"No, you can't do that. We'll find a way out of this mess. Even with your statement, the police still have to prove their case. I could have lied to you," I explained.

"I've got it! You need just one person to lie for you and say you told them you didn't give your mother the morphine overdose."

"It's a big thing to ask people to perjure themselves in court. They could go to jail… It's hard enough for me to do it. I can't ask someone else to sell their soul. Besides they have already interviewed everyone, so they can't suddenly remember some crucial piece of information and change their statements."

"No one wants you to go to jail, Sean. There'll be someone who won't hesitate to do it," he said.

"Forget it Ian."

"I've got it, the perfect person!" Ian exclaimed. "Your sister! Jo! She hasn't been interviewed yet. She's stable, intelligent, beautiful, and a mother. Of course she'll say you told her you didn't do it. She'll do anything to keep you out of jail."

"I don't know, Ian. Jo has been my savior since I was a toddler, but I don't think I can ask her to break the law, and I'm not certain that she would if I did."

"Just tell her that it'll really piss off Mary," Ian said. "She'll do it."

Monday 4 October 2010

I arrived here with only a small travel bag of clothes to last the conference, so today I did the rounds of the discount shops. The main thing was gym and pool gear so I can get into my normal exercise routine. Normal? Nothing will be normal here.

Since I might be here for a while, I needed an EFTPOS card, and I had to change my address.

"Are you the guy in the paper?" asked the bank clerk.

Where normally I would have ducked and dived such a conversation and then bolted for the door, today I launched straight into an explanation of why I'm here. Now there's nothing to hide, as my life could be laid bare to the world in the court case. Besides, I need all the support I can get. Perhaps this lady will tell her husband that she met the man accused of murdering his mother, then he may tell a friend and another friend ... and, who knows, there may be a member of the jury at the end of this chain, who might be more sympathetic.

I then had a strong black Americano at Starbucks. While I hate supporting them, at least I'm guaranteed a perfect mug every time. After that I popped by Jindra's place. I felt strong enough to take some more punishment, along with her insightful advice.

"You're a fool Sean, a complete fool," she began.

"Why this time?"

"You should be putting your family first. Those boys are growing up without you. You should never have come back."

"But I am putting my family first. If I hadn't come back to New Zealand to sort this out now, then I wouldn't be able to come back here, ever. I would be arrested on landing in New Zealand – in front of my sons, Jindra."

"But you have an English passport. You can go to England or Australia."

"They have extradition treaties with New Zealand. I have to sort this out now or be trapped in South Africa for life."

"Then bring Raine here. You are going to jail. Your family needs to be here to visit you."

"I'm not going to jail, Jindra."

"But you are a fool," she said. "You showed the same confidence two weeks ago when you said you wouldn't be arrested, and now look at the mess you're in." It's true. I did say this to Jindra when I first got back to Dunedin.

"Well, I know I won't be found guilty."

"You will be. A friend of mine is a high-ranking judge in Auckland, and she says you're in big trouble and she thinks you will definitely go to jail."

"She hasn't heard the evidence. She can't possibly say that."

"She has followed the story in the newspaper."

"I rest my case."

Tuesday 5 October 2010

I went for my first gym workout today. The physical and mental focus of a gym session feels like total solitude, no matter how many pulsating bodies surround me.

When I phoned Detective Rowley afterwards, she told me the laptop wasn't ready yet, but definitely would be by tomorrow. Sometimes I wonder if they're toying with me. How long can it take to copy a laptop hard drive? They've had it eleven days now. She said they have to make another copy. How many copies do they need?

Later the same night

I've spoken to Raine and she shares my confidence that I'll get off. Each phone call we discuss different aspects of my manuscript and how it could be open to interpretation. She's enjoying the challenge of assisting with my defense and untangling the riddles of words I use. She seems to be spending hours on it each day.

Wednesday 6 October 2010

Finally, I've got my laptop back. When I picked it up, Detective Rowley asked if she could have the PIN number to my South African cell phone SIM card. What do they take me for? But it's good to have the laptop again. I phoned Ian to tell him the good news.

The Last Waltz: Love, Death & Betrayal

"I better tell you some more bad news I learnt from my teacher workshop notes," he said. "The police may have added spyware to your laptop, which means they'll have a team of experts at the station analyzing everything you write on the computer. They can detect each key you type, as you type it."

"Good grief, that seems a bit excessive."

"They will have accessed all the emails you've sent from that laptop, no matter how long ago," he said.

"Damn, my computer is a smoking gun!"

Len just phoned. He said the police have given him the evidence against me. He said I'd better see him straight away.

Straight away. Doesn't sound like good news.

Later the same day

"Right, Sean, they've handed me the first part of the evidence against you. There's more coming, but probably nothing as damning as this. I've gone through it very quickly. Who is this guy Mr. Landreth? He appears to be their key witness."

"That's my oldest friend, Ian Landreth. But he's on our side."

"Well, he's dumped you in it. He says you confessed to him. Are you sure it's the same person? Mr. Landreth has given a very detailed statement, in fact seventeen pages of it. He says you told him the day after your mother died that you gave her an overdose of crushed morphine tablets."

"No, he didn't mean it. He's going to tell the court I didn't tell him anything."

"Too late now, it's in writing." Len said. "He's their key witness."

"Can he retract his statement?"

"He can, but they can still read out the original in court."

"This is a mess."

"Your friend Jindra Tichy also hasn't helped you," he added.

"Not possible. She's my other best friend."

The Last Waltz: Love, Death & Betrayal

"Unusual friends." Anyway, I'll let you go through Jindra Tichy's statement on your own, since I haven't had time yet to study all of the private emails you exchanged with her. Of course the police have studied all of them."

Len also told me that the police disclosed, from the time they first knocked on my motel door, that I've been under constant surveillance, with a detective following my every move, including when I retrieved the rubbish I put in a bin the morning of my arrest. This rubbish was the paperwork related to my manuscript, and apparently they are using it as an argument that I was trying to impede their investigation by destroying evidence.

As a consequence of their surveillance, they obtained a post office video recording in order to ascertain the address I had written on a package I posted to Wellington. Detective Verry had even flown to Wellington to find out what was in the package, obviously thinking it was some evidence I wanted rid of. He would have been very disappointed when he got to the house of my friend, Chris Walker, to find it was a cell phone charger. The reason for that is a long story. This is very unsettling. I wonder how many days they spent following me. This information strongly suggests that they bugged my motel phone and have put spyware on my computer. I feel so violated.

Oh well, there's nothing I can do now – except wring Ian's neck... and Jindra's?

Thursday 7 October 2010

Jo hasn't got back to me yet. I've left her several messages to call me before the police get to her. I'm still not sure if I can ask her to lie to them. It's just not right, but I'm going to do it. Oh God, what would Mum think of me?

I need to keep calm and carry on. It's okay. I've got to stay focused. Mum wouldn't want me in jail for murdering her. I must keep going down this dreadful path of deception. I can't doubt myself. I just wish I didn't have to drag others into this terrible hell with me.

"Cheer up, Sean. You realize you're going to be here for the Dunedin summer?"

The Last Waltz: Love, Death & Betrayal

"That's a token of comfort. Thanks, Ian."

"Yes indeed: summer, autumn, the winter, and maybe next summer too."

Friday 8 October 2010

Fantastic news! Len said today that he thinks my case shouldn't go to court. He says it's madness if they prosecute me for a work of fiction, and that I must give an interview to the police and tell them the whole story. He said since I was the only person present at my mother's death, if I say I didn't do it then there should be no case to answer to.

Len said that although it's not guaranteed, there is a chance that if I make this statement, they may drop the charges. He added that it's very unusual for a lawyer to offer their client up on a platter to the prosecution, but I'm so convincing it's worth a go.

He then drafted a letter to the police stating that the manuscript was fiction and requested that they interview me. He told me that they would probably want me to make a public statement denying that I assisted in my mother's suicide. Finally, some hope. Perhaps I can get home soon.

Later that night

Hell. Several emails from my university today. It's their Friday morning and there's a reporter from the South African *Sunday Times* snooping around, asking questions about my arrest. What makes it really bad news is that I've hardly told anyone in South Africa about it, which my employers must interpret as showing incredible disrespect.

Why didn't I tell them? Maybe Jindra's right and I am a damn fool. I've been living in cloud cuckoo land, hoping the whole thing would disappear before there was a need to own up to it. Perhaps I didn't have the courage to tell them – to try to explain why I've been charged with attempting to murder my mother.

Damn it, I can just imagine their reaction. I was stupid, of course. It was only a matter of time before a student or staff member stumbled across my arrest on the web. Yeah, stupid... It's easy to see it's stupid once it's too late to change what I've said/done.

Now I must swing into damage control before the story appears in the *Sunday Times*. Tonight I'll email the vice-chancellor and dean to explain myself, and some explanation that will be. They didn't even know about my book, let alone my mother's death.

Saturday 9 October 2010

My lab's manager, Eugenia, just called on Skype. She's the only university colleague that I've informed about my situation. She thinks a story in the *Sunday Times* will not get too much attention and will blow over quickly, but I should send a low-key email to all staff and postgraduate students in the department to explain to them what's happened. She said I don't need to worry about the lab as she's got everything under control for now.

Sunday 10 October 2010

Tonight I had dinner at Jindra's place, and she said Len Andersen had handled her divorce and charged $6000 (R30 000) Hmmm. I don't think I've found the cheapest lawyer in Dunedin. I've heard several times that lawyers charged in six-minute segments of $30.

Last time I saw him, Len made me a cup of coffee, and it took about six minutes. That's a $30 cuppa, and it was weak and tepid (though at that price I could hardly send it back).

Later same night

"PROFESSOR ARRESTED IN NEW ZEALAND FOR MERCY KILLING"

What on earth? Raine has just phoned with the sensational news that this is the banner headline across the front page of the South African *Sunday Times*. While we spoke, she measured the headline with her hand.

"It's two hand widths high" she said.

"I'm glad you've got small hands."

"And the article covers most of the front page, with follow-up articles on page six that cover the whole page," she said. "I checked the paper readership online, and it's 3.5 million!"

"It doesn't make sense. There's no story at all. Is South Africa as crazy as New Zealand? How could this get such attention? I was arrested in New Zealand for committing a crime in New Zealand, and this was four years ago. What's the big deal?"

"But don't worry, they're very supportive articles."

What worries me now is that it will provoke the New Zealand police into thinking I'm letting it out in South Africa deliberately to get public support in New Zealand, since the media are gagged here. At least it doesn't reveal my plan to say the manuscript is fiction.

I hate all of this. I feel sick thinking about it.

Monday 11 October 2010

Things are turning to custard. Following yesterday's sensational *Sunday Times* story, the media are all over my campus in Cape Town. Apparently, they camped outside the biotechnology department most of today, asking students if they know me and what kind of person am I, and for any bits of gossip. They've also interviewed the vice-chancellor and the dean.

Jeepers, I wonder what the students will say about me behind my back.

I've spoken to Eugenia, who says the whole university seems to be abuzz with my story, and copies of the *Sunday Times* are circulating around the campus. She will meet the lab students tomorrow to calm them about my possible internment. That won't go down well.

Oh, hell. Hell.

Later the same day

Ross Creek Reservoir is beautiful and peaceful, such a tranquil spot: not a breath of wind, and the native bush and sky are reflected perfectly on the water as birds call to each other. It's one of my favorite places in Dunedin.

My calmness is not from peace, but from having the stuffing completely knocked out of me. I feel nothing worse can happen. Every phone call from a policeman, journalist, or lawyer brings more bad news, but I'm so stunned I've become impervious to shock and feel nothing.

I know I can't sink any lower, and that this isn't such a bad place to be.

Tuesday 12 October 2010

Text message from Jo: *Sori, couldn't get hold of U as U asked. Just had 2 hr. interview with police.*

I don't know whether to feel relief or disappointment. I just needed one person to lie for me. I told her to let me know before she had her interview so I could prepare her. We didn't talk earlier because I thought the police may be monitoring my calls. I still can't get her on the phone. But perhaps this is a good thing. I'm steadily destroying my own soul, and I can't take my sister with me.

Why are the police continuing their investigation so long after my arrest? They've got heaps on me already. Len tells me the police haven't responded to his request for an interview. Once again my heart sinks. Perhaps they don't want to talk to me because they have enough evidence to convict me. I guess they're pretty pissed off because I refused to be interviewed when they first took me in. That means I could be stuck here until my trial in June next year – and then sent to jail.

It's all too much.

Later the same day

I popped around to Ian's place to pick up a soft mattress. I commented that John's mattress was like concrete.

"Get used to it, Sean," he said.

I had a quiet night at John's. It's comforting to be with a simple, decent guy who has no airs or graces, but is the salt of the earth. I've noticed he focuses on the small details of life around him, quite a rare characteristic. I asked Ian about this, and he said even when they were kids, John was always doing jigsaw puzzles and would complete difficult ones in a few hours, when other people took a few days. He has also developed an interest in making model planes and boats, and tonight I felt at peace watching him carefully assembling the *Bismarck*.

Wednesday 13 October 2010

Bail signing today. It's so degrading. To ease the humiliation, I joked with the elderly woman officer.

"I skipped the country for a week, but I'm back!"

"I know you wouldn't do that dear," she said. "I would love to chat with you personally, but you know how it is with the law."

Yeah, I know how it is with the law. I just wish the politicians would show some courage and change the law. There are many people out there in similar situations to the one I'm in – and we aren't criminals.

After bail signing, I always have a feeling of euphoria - it's as if I've just written an exam. It's hard to understand why. I think it's because of my fear of the consequences of forgetting to sign in, and the relief that I remembered. A missed signing leads directly to jail. The problem is that every day feels the same, and I really fear a Wednesday could come and go without me noticing.

Later the same day

I am preparing myself in case the police agree to interview me. I'm ready to tell them the manuscript was embellished to sell to a publisher.

When you're not telling the truth you have to draw a line, but where do I draw the line? Where does the truth stop and the fiction begin? Sometimes I'm lying, sometimes I'm not. It's a terrible tangle.

It's so unfair that I'm in the situation of having to lie to the police and then weigh up how many lies to tell them.

The Last Waltz: Love, Death & Betrayal

The worst part of all is that if I lie and claim the entire description of mum's death is fabricated, it is a denial of her courage, and of a deed I'm not ashamed of. But if I tell the truth, I will lose my job, and worse, I'll be tagged a murderer for the rest of my life, and my children's lives. Is there a compromise?

It is so unreal contemplating how many lies to tell the police when all of my life I've tried to live by truth and honesty. It's like a bad dream, a nightmare. I'm in a place I should never have landed in and I wish I could awaken from it.

Thursday 14 October 2010

Will it never end?

Mary's ex-husband Richard phoned to say that the police are coming up to Wellington to interview him on Monday. I have to accept the fact that this will go on and on.

I finally got hold of Jo on the landline. (Cell phones don't feature prominently in her life.) She said she told the police I'd never confided in her about what I'd done, and the detective was surprised since, from reading the manuscript, he knew we were very close.

In her statement she said two years prior to Mum's death, when she visited her in hospital after a cancer operation, Mum asked her to go home and get her some pills she had hidden away just in case things went wrong. She said it was a known fact that Mum always kept a little stockpile, "just in case."

Off the record, the detective said that he didn't believe that I should be before the courts, showing sympathy for the situation I'd been in with Mum. Jo asked him why they were wasting so much time and so many resources on this case, and he said they had no choice but to follow up when a law was broken. Jo thought the report he wrote up would be slanted in my favor.

The Last Waltz: Love, Death & Betrayal

Later the same day

I'm desperate to get back to South Africa and be with Raine and the boys.

The police are dragging out their investigation. Len thinks it will be months before it gets committed to the high court and the trial could be late next year. He said these trials were often repeatedly delayed and it could take years before they came to a conclusion.

I can't wait here for years, even to be found not guilty. I think I must do the unthinkable: plead guilty now and go straight to sentencing. What's the worst that can happen? Lesley Martin, who injected her terminally ill mother with morphine, was sentenced to fifteen months and spent eight months in prison before being paroled.

I'll probably get less than that for pleading guilty early. Surely I'll be back in Cape Town after six months in prison. I don't feel I have a choice. I have to think of my family.

I've just phoned Raine and put my plan to her. She is stunned.

Friday 15 October 2010

Raine says she didn't sleep at all after I spoke to her.

She doesn't want me to plead guilty, even if it gets me home sooner. Even pleading guilty to a lesser charge of assisted suicide isn't right, she says. Her parents are appalled at the idea. Her father told her to tell me that I didn't need to rush home, that everything would be fine – he's looking after the garden, the dogs, the pool and cooking – and I shouldn't feel a need to come back.

They all said it was important that I be found not guilty and not go to jail, because then I wouldn't be able to talk to them every day and would just disappear for a year, which would be terrible for all of them. And it could cost me my job.

Raine said that she'd been in shock all day and felt like she had a stone on her heart. She blames Mary and wants to get even by telling everyone that Mary caused this. Raine often mentions Mary and how absolutely certain she is that

Mary's behind our misery, even though the evidence is only circumstantial – and Raine has never met her. She says that Mary was so angry at my resisting her attempts to stop publication that she's the only person with a strong enough motive to want to bring me down. Her argument is sound and I can't imagine who else could be behind this, but I still give Mary the benefit of the doubt. She's not a monster. She's my sister and always will be.

I've made up my mind to go with their decision and plead not guilty. I feel it is as much the family's decision as mine. At least there's certainty about something.

So what now? I'm just sitting around contemplating the story I'll tell the police. It does seem, just like a story, and that everything is a deception. I was the only person present at my mother's death, so I'm the only person who actually knows how she died, and whatever I say has to be given a lot of credence.

For the jury, it will surely come down to my credibility:

Does this man have integrity? Would he lie under oath?

Under oath. I never really thought about it like that. Would I lie under oath? I don't believe in the Bible, but I believe in the principles of honesty it represents, which are the foundation of our society. If I put my hand on it and swear to tell the truth, and then lie, what kind of person am I?

I feel like I'm climbing down a ladder, rung by rung, lie by lie, into a deep dark hole.

Saturday 16 October 2010

"Do you want a cup of tea, Sean?" Len asked.
"No, I'm good, thanks."
"Are you sure? I'm having one."
"Definitely not, thanks."

I've just received his first bill, for the few days when he read my book.

"I had to come to work on a Saturday to work on your case."

"I'm sorry about that."

I'm sure he charges time and a half on the weekend.

"The police have sent me a fax requesting that your pre-committal hearing be delayed a month until 17 December because they need more time to prepare the prosecution case."

"Another delay. No, that's not fair."

"I agree. This request has to go to the court, and I hope the judge will also agree. I'm going to say they can have the extra time if they let you return to South Africa until the trial," Len said. "But don't raise your hopes, since it's a big issue that New Zealand doesn't have an extradition treaty with South Africa."

Ross Creek reservoir: later

How much longer must I wait here? This could drag on for months or even years. I thought I had reached rock bottom, but I keep finding new depths, and I feel gutted – powerless. I've got to do something to take control of my life, my circumstances.

Later that night

I have a plan.

After Ross Creek I paid a visit to Peter Hinds, one of Mum's dearest friends, to ask for his help. Shortly after I got there, Vivienne arrived, and we sat around the table in his dimly lit dining room. There was an air of uncertainty, as I'd earlier let Peter know I had something to tell him, and he deduced it had to be something serious, especially so late at night. Even Vivienne looked far from comfortable.

"So what did you have to tell me, Sean?" he asked, once we got past the small talk. He anticipated bad news.

"I was wondering if you could do me a small favor, please." I saw Peter's face muscles tighten. He has supported me throughout, both as a friend and because of his commitment to the euthanasia cause, but at the same time, he is fearful of the law.

The Last Waltz: Love, Death & Betrayal

"I need to get Raine to post me my British passport, just in case I have to make an emergency dash back to South Africa. I don't want the police to find out and confiscate it. Do you mind if she posts it to you, please?"

Peter grimaced again.

"Won't my address be too risky, since they know you were staying here?" he sidestepped. "Perhaps they're monitoring the mail to my house."

This seemed extremely unlikely, but he had a point. I paused, sensing Vivienne's sympathy and hoping she might suggest her place. "Yes, I suppose you're right, Peter." I didn't want him to feel cornered. "But the envelope will be addressed to you."

"It would still have a South African stamp," he said. That was enough for me. I knew it was time to back off.

There was a long, uncomfortable pause. Vivienne was searching her conscience. As a woman of God, she couldn't desert me. "You could use my address. They would never connect us."

"Not at all, Vivienne," Peter interrupted. "They'll have connected you with me and they'll be watching your post too." Peter is a man of considerable honor and he would never let his woman be sacrificed ahead of him. "If you want to take a chance with my place, that's fine."

Now I was feeling terrible. Although they had both offered the use of their addresses, they had succumbed under pressure. I thanked them and told them I would think about it, as there was no real hurry. As I was leaving, Vivienne discreetly slipped me a piece of paper with her address written on it. She would sleep peacefully tonight.

Later that night

I'm going to do it. I've made up my mind to skip the country. I'll come back for the trial in June, but for now I can't take any more of this. However, I can't tell Raine the truth.

"Please get my British passport in the post tomorrow. I'd better have it ready just in case there's an emergency with you or the boys," I told her, trying not to show any desperation. I was calling from a public telephone because I couldn't take any chances with the police monitoring my computer and landline.

"But why do you want it now? Can't I courier it when you need it?" she asked.

"If there's an emergency there won't be time for you to send it. I'll need to jump on a plane immediately." It doesn't feel good to be deceiving her, but I can't tell her my plan, for as much as she wants me back, she's too rational to encourage me to evade the law. She certainly won't post the passport if she knows.

"Okay, but what happens if the police catch you with it?" Her logical mind was working overtime.

"They mustn't or I'll go to jail, as that would be a breach of my bail conditions. I was instructed to hand over all my passports."

"I think it's too risky, then."

"It'll be okay. Just do it, please. Post it to Vivienne's address – the police certainly won't be monitoring her mail – and once I have it I'll immediately hide it in another house. There's no real risk."

"So long as you don't use it."

"Of course not."

Monday 18 October 2010

Oh no. I've just seen Len, and the police are definitely refusing to interview me. They obviously think they have a cut-and-dry case and there's no need. So he's decided I am to write an affidavit stating that I did not assist my mother to her death and that my manuscript was a work of fiction. He said that he would submit this to the court and the judge may well toss the case out. He said the police have a very weak case, since I was the only person present when my mother died, and I'm prepared to declare under oath that I didn't do anything.

He said there was every chance I could be home by Christmas, a free man.

The Last Waltz: Love, Death & Betrayal

Tuesday 19 October 2010

I had a terrible night's sleep.

Mum's death is only known by me. No one can ever be sure what happened that night. Surely any normal human being would do all he could to be free, to protect his family and their livelihood? It's only one lie.

Today Len wants me to sign the affidavit. It is time to commit myself to my lies, but I'm struggling with it. I'm not a liar and what I did for Mum is not a crime.

If I deny helping my mother to die, I am giving up on the principle that it was the right thing to do. To deny it happened is like saying it was wrong. It's also dishonoring my mother, what she did and what I did. It is selling my soul. This is a moral decision. It should have nothing to do with family, money, and future prospects. My integrity is the only thing I own in this life.

I need more time to think. I phoned Len and told him I couldn't see him today. I told him I had important stuff to prepare for my work. More lies. I have some searching to do. I can't ask anyone now. I've talked enough. This decision is about my soul.

Wednesday 20 October 2010
Ross Creek Reservoir

It was getting dark and the stars were out. I kept staring into the night, looking for a miracle. The life I once knew is gone. Her death has left my life in ruins, and my soul is lost and confused.

Can she see me now? I close my eyes. I know she is out there somewhere.

"Why don't you answer? I have so many questions I need answers to."

\Later that night

She's out there. I can feel her in the sky. I am waiting. The sky is waiting. I am open to her. The time has come. Will she turn away?

The Last Waltz: Love, Death & Betrayal

And then I heard her. The message was so simple and so pure: "No more lies. No more lies."

Thursday 21 October 2010

I slept beautifully, and now I understand. The truth sets you free. I will probably go to jail as Lesley Martin did, but at least I will be free.

But truth comes at a price, and now I have to deal with its consequences. First, I have to tell Len, who won't be happy about my deception. Perhaps he'll drop the case. Who cares? I'm free!

I will write a full and honest statement. My confession will prevent a high court trial and the likely media frenzy, and it will save so many people, especially those who were going to commit perjury in court to protect me. At last there's an end to that.

I'll probably go straight to sentencing now, and be given a chance to show remorse for the "crime" I committed in exchange for a more lenient sentence. But I won't do that. I don't regret what I did; I only regret that I had to do what I did.

I can't tell Raine what I'm doing. She'll be devastated. She would never understand my principled position, and why should she? She is a mother with two young babies and a struggling business. Each day for her is a fight for survival, and she wants me back as a pillar of the family, not sacrificing myself for the sake of principles she can't understand. I keep reassuring her that I will lie until the very end.

Yet I must draw the line – a line that defines my existence, my integrity and my humanness.

Later the same day

Len stared at me in disbelief. A week ago he was in awe of my command of the law and convinced of my innocence. Now he saw a liar, although one relieved at discovering the core of his existence.

The Last Waltz: Love, Death & Betrayal

"It's okay, Sean, it's not the first time I've had a client change their testimony," he said after some thought. "Have you told me the complete story now?"

"Yes, I'm being totally honest with you," I replied. "And I don't think it should be referred to as a story now."

"No, of course not."

"I want to tell the truth and plead guilty to assisted suicide. I want them to withdraw the attempted murder charge. I want to be free and..."

"Not so fast." he interrupted. "The prosecution cannot prove how your mother died. She could have died from natural causes."

"I don't understand."

"You should not plead guilty to assisted suicide. You thought you were giving her a lethal dose, but how did you know what was a lethal dose? And how do you know what you gave her actually killed her?"

"So I can tell the truth and still be found not guilty?"

"Yes, indeed."

This is wonderful news. I hugged Len. He seemed a bit uncomfortable, but I was in a hugging mood.

I can confess to giving my mother what I thought was a lethal overdose and still be found not guilty. Raine will be very happy to hear this, but there's no need to tell her of my planned confession until the actual trial. She insists I don't admit to doing anything, so why should I put her under stress for so long when I'm so far away?

Len is submitting an application for a change of my bail conditions to allow me to return to South Africa until the trial.

It is miserably cold, with snow to low levels on the hills around Dunedin. I have no job here, no family, no normal life, but I feel so good. I am a new man today.

I updated Ian on today's developments.

"Let me get this straight. You're going to tell the complete truth?"

"Yes."

"Like I told the truth."

"Yes."

"And felt like shit."

The Last Waltz: Love, Death & Betrayal

Saturday 23 October 2010

Brother Fergus in London emailed saying the police in Dunedin had phoned him and asked if he would make himself available for an interview. Now I'm getting wise to the police and know that when they ask for an interview it's going to be very soon – probably to stop the accused from interfering with the witness!

Monday 25 October 2010

What an amazing blessing! Archbishop Desmond Tutu has written to the court requesting that I be granted bail to return to my family in South Africa. He gives his assurance that I will return to New Zealand to stand trial. This is an extraordinary act of kindness, since he hardly knows me. He is the chancellor of my university, but I've only met him a few times in passing. How could the court refuse such a request!

Tuesday 26 October 2010

Oh bugger. I got a call from Len.

"I've done some research into legal precedents, and it's not as simple as I thought. Based on the interpretation of the law, if you admit to giving your mother an overdose, you're admitting attempted murder."

"That's nonsense. Mum begged me for it," I said.

"That's the law, I'm afraid. However, they still have to prove that what you gave her was a lethal dose, so you can still enter a not guilty plea," he explained. "But please be careful who you speak to about your case, and say nothing to the media."

"Okay. Don't worry, I haven't spoken to any reporters. But I do want people to know why I did what I did for my mother."

"I understand that, but you'll get your day in court." Len reassured me. "By the way, the police have now handed over an interview with Chris Catley, and her evidence is quite contrary to the rest."

"I know. I'll speak to her."
"No don't do that, you shouldn't speak to witnesses."
"But she's my friend."
"Yep, that much is very clear."

Wednesday 27 October 2010

Things are looking up. Len phoned again today to say the judge had granted me bail to return home. Fantastic news! Skipping the country wasn't really my style. The only catch is that I can't leave until mid-December for various legal reasons. I phoned Raine straight away, and she said she can live with the delay so long as I'm coming back. I emailed Archbishop Tutu. There's no doubt that his assurance convinced the judge.

There is another little catch. I need three people to put up surety of $30,000 each. They don't have to hand over the money, just the copy of their home title deeds, so if I don't come back for the trial the court can seize their houses. I can't see it being a problem finding three people, as I have several friends here who are well established in life. It's not as if I'm going to run away.

I visited the police station to sign my bail form today and to be greeted by the same woman officer.

"Hi Sean, good to see you. Just sign right here."

I signed the form as usual.

"Thanks for popping in and we'll see you next week."

Like going to the corner shop to get my Sunday newspaper.

Sunday 12 December 2010 (five weeks later)

Only a week to go now. I fear the media attention that may be waiting for me. There have been several big headlines in South Africa in recent weeks:

"TUTU FREES MERCY KILLER"
"A WIFE'S ANGUISH"
"MERCY KILLER COMING HOME"

The Last Waltz: Love, Death & Betrayal

Although I'm not comfortable in the spotlight, I now appreciate how much the media have helped Raine. The regular newspaper articles have engaged the public in my story and won their support. This has helped Raine tremendously. She was feeling very alone and depressed, but now she's surrounded by well-wishers excited about what will happen next.

Since the New Zealand media aren't allowed to report on my story, I'm going to feed them something they are allowed to publish. The objective is to get my name out there as someone other than a mother-killer. This is the only way the jury can be made to understand who I really am before my image is clouded in the trial. Today I contacted the *Otago Daily Times* offering my services to the New Zealand Defense Force to identify the bodies in a mass grave recently found in Japan. The grave is presumed to contain New Zealand coastguards killed during World War II. The reporter was bursting with enthusiasm to get this into print.

Monday 13 December 2010

Here comes trouble.

The Dunedin police flew to Auckland to interview my publisher Chris Catley again today, and she was questioned for three and a half hours. When I learnt they were on their way up, I immediately phoned and told her to tell the truth and admit that she received the original manuscript. If she keeps trying to cover for me they will charge her with perjury, but I don't think she's going to budge.

"How many times must I tell you Sean, I stand by my authors," she said.

I immediately told Len what was happening.

"Leave her, Sean. Chris Catley must look after Chris Catley."

I stand by my friends – and yet I'm supposed to let Chris, Dame Chris, go down for perjury?

My publisher can be very stubborn. She took on my sister and her lawyers in the battle to stop the publication of my book, and reveled in the drama. Chris Catley is 84 years old and was recently awarded a dame-hood by the Queen for her services to publishing and journalism. I'm sure any other publisher would have been scared off by threats of legal action – but Chris Catley, DAME Chris Catley, didn't flinch. You don't get a dame-hood by being intimated by big sisters! Mary made a big mistake in taking on Chris. She was also dying from cancer. But she's such a strong person, she would have scared the police!!!

Later the same day

This afternoon we gathered at the high court for the signing of surety so I can leave the country. Peter Hinds and Ian arrived at about the same time, and Peter, who seemed a bit nervous about the whole thing, signed first. I don't blame him, as it was quite a big deal to put his house up when he'd only known me a relatively short time.

Ian then approached the counter.

"If Sean dies before he returns, do I lose my house?" he asked the court registrar.

While we were there, Detective Verry spotted us and came and chatted. It was like bringing old friends together when I introduced him to Ian and Peter. He clearly wanted to help me and warned me about speaking to the media in South Africa. He also mentioned that there had been eight detectives on my case.

"That's good for your book sales," Ian whispered. "I wonder if they had a book club."

Tonight I booked my ticket to return to Cape Town. Not long now.

Later the same day

Len told me that the police documents he's just received indicate that Mary refused to be interviewed. This doesn't make sense at all, as it leaves unexplained how the police came to be in possession of her manuscript. I can't think of any logical explanation for this. Len also said that the police recently searched Mum's house in Broad Bay. Come on! What are they thinking? Are they looking for the murder weapon, the mortar and pestle?

The Last Waltz: Love, Death & Betrayal

Wednesday 15 December 2010

I just got a call from Len to let me know that the police have executed another three search warrants, two on media houses and the other on the pharmacy where I collected Mum's morphine prescription. They're not letting up.

I signed bail for the last time. What a pleasure!

Sunday 19 December 2010

I have decided to found a new organization called DignitySA to seek a law change on voluntary euthanasia in South Africa. I've already pulled a few supporters together in South Africa to get things moving. The first thing they asked me to do was to get a media liaison person. I asked Kate Cane, an old friend of mine, if she could do it. She is very keen and has already arranged a press conference for the day after I get back to Cape Town! I will have to think carefully about doing this in the light of Detective Verry's advice, but she is insisting it has to be that day because the media wants the news fresh. My supporters are also insistent that this is needed to kick-start the organization. I've felt so harassed these past months. Campaigning for a law change will certainly let them know they can't walk all over me.

I'm off today: Dunedin to Christchurch, Christchurch to Sydney, Sydney to Singapore, Singapore to Johannesburg, Johannesburg to Cape Town. A total of 36 hours travelling time without a significant stop – and when I get there, a news conference the following morning. What madness!

SOUTH AFRICA

December 2010 to October 2011

I've been in S.A. for nearly 1 year. I did give that press conference the day after I returned to Cape Town, and I shared it with the university Vice-Chancellor and Deputy Vic-Chancellor. Although I was warned not to speak to the media, this was definitely the right thing to do. The

The Last Waltz: Love, Death & Betrayal

conference demonstrated that the university supported me, and were not just standing beside me because I was "innocent until proven guilty." Rather, it supported my decision to help my Mum die. The Vice Chancellor even told the press that he would have done the same thing in the same circumstances. Of course the irony of this is that I haven't admitted it! I have said nothing since my arrest.

Because there was so much media publicity in South Africa after my arrest, the media and the public assumed I had helped my mother die, and almost without exception strongly supported my presumed actions. Following that press conference, there were several weeks of saturation coverage of my story in all forms of media. In fact, my story was rated the biggest end-of-year news story in the country. This is extraordinary, in a country gripped in terrible and tragic news stories day after day. I suspect that my story appealed to the media and the public because many people empathized with the situation I was in.

Of course the media coverage was totally against the advice of my lawyer and the police in New Zealand, and it was hardly surprising when the prosecutors in New Zealand called for a special hearing with the judge, demanding my bail be revoked and I be ordered to return to New Zealand. The prosecutors claimed I was manipulating the media in South Africa to influence the jury in New Zealand (I admit it had crossed my mind!). They said I was getting a lot of coverage on the Internet, which I wouldn't have if the court had kept me in New Zealand. They saw it as a breach of trust... Fortunately, the judge didn't see it that way.

During these past eight months I have changed lawyers, from Len to Roger. Once Roger assured me that if I hired him the government's Legal Aid would cover all my costs, and I would never have to pay it back, it was obvious I had to sack Len.

Roger is considered one of the top criminal lawyers in the country, and has been very good at keeping me informed of every development. He explained to me what everyone wanted to know – why was I charged with "attempted murder." He said the police had charged me with this instead of assisted suicide, because attempted murder is easier to prove. In attempted murder, they have to show only that an attempt was made to end a life, and they don't have to prove the cause of death; whereas, assisted suicide is a wider-ranging charge in which they do have to prove cause of death.

The trial date was delayed a few times. Eventually, a date of 25th October was offered, and I was warned that if I didn't accept this date the trial could be delayed another year. The date – 25 October – is the very day Mum died. Did they do this deliberately to upset me? If so, it's working...

My dear friend Jindra has been persistent with her advice, always meaning well, but often totally out of touch with reality. Last night she phoned insisting I don't come back for the trial... I now understand why she didn't put her house up for bail surety!

Last week I went to visit Archbishop Tutu. He is awe-inspiring - every moment with him feels sacred. We have met a few times at the university, but then I was just another professor. Now I feel I have a connection with him. He made the effort to write to the New Zealand court, to guarantee that I would return to New Zealand to stand trial. And he did this when he hardly knew me. This alone is a measure of the man, to show trust in someone is to encourage trust. I still can't believe this man put his name on the line to guarantee I would return to New Zealand.

As I left his room, he embraced me and whispered in my ear, "I hope you will return to your trial in New Zealand, Sean."

"What! Sorry, Archbishop, what did you say?"

"I said, I hope all will go well for your trial in New Zealand, Sean."

NEW ZEALAND

Tuesday 11 October 2011: 14 days until trial

It's two weeks to the trial. Time is dragging. I just want to get on with it.

There's been an interesting development: Roger noticed that the police have prepared a summary of Fergus's original

The Last Waltz: Love, Death & Betrayal

statement with a couple of new sentences inserted into it. These sentences slant it to make it seem that Fergus thinks I'm on a crusade to change the law, and everything I do is related to that in an attempt to taint the jury's impression of me. He told me to ask Fergus to check the summary statement carefully before he signs it.

I phoned Fergus straight away.

"Yes, a steely looking chap brought the summary to my house to sign. I'm glad they didn't expect me to travel all the way to the New Zealand House again," he said.

"Did you check to see if they had inserted extra lines before you signed?" I asked. "My lawyer thinks they did."

"It seems much the same." Fergus said. "According to the policeman, they only want me to say the manuscript is true."

"But 'much the same' isn't good enough. You should have checked the statement."

"Why?" He sounded genuinely surprised.

"That's just the way it is, Fergus. They want a conviction and will do whatever it takes."

"Ohhh."

I gave Fergus a rundown on what he should say in his evidence. Initially, I didn't want to go this route because the prosecutor may ask him if I had given him instructions. However, now I feel there's no choice because, as the only family member giving evidence, his point of view is crucial. I told him to say how close I was to Mum, and in particular that helping her had nothing to do with a cause. My God, I can't have the prosecutor painting me as a campaigner and not a doting son.

It's a great shame that Jo is in China and we can't even set up a video link so that she can testify. I really need her here.

Roger wants me to visit him in Hamilton because he doesn't like the idea of us meeting for the first time in Dunedin the day before the trial. It sort of makes sense, but I don't feel like being a guest in his house at this time.

On the phone today he warned me that once the trial starts, I will be in custody, and I'll have to report to the court thirty minutes before the trial begins. I'll be kept in a police holding cell whenever the court is not in session. Evidently this is to prevent me from bumping into jury members or witnesses. He also said that at the end of each day he will apply for me to be granted bail to return home. He was pretty shocked when I told him I might stay in a caravan park during the trial, until I explained that I would need to be alone during this time to quietly assimilate and reflect on the day's events. He said he understood, because he would feel the same way.

Thursday 13 October 2011: 12 days until trial

I'm at Roger's place in Hamilton. What a day! I'm not sure what to make of Roger. I'd say his defining characteristic, as an instinctive peacemaker, is to want all things for all people. It's a charming trait and reminds me of others I know, but the problem with "yes" people is that they usually end up pissing off everyone.

We went over some of the evidence today, and if I showed the slightest concern about anything, Roger was quick to respond in a calm, reassuring voice: "I really don't think that will be a problem." I lost track of how many times he said that.

Roger made a point of telling me that his services would cost about R210,000. It's not a subject I'm comfortable discussing, but it was reasonable for him to bring up the matter at our first meeting. I don't think my case, for Roger, is about money. At least he succeeded in getting me a legal aid loan. The irony is that if Len Andersen had thought of this option, he could have offered it to me when this nightmare began.

I found out why Roger wants me here. He insists that I must not take the stand.

"Your case is extremely complex and interesting," he said. "I need to keep sowing doubt in the jurors' minds, so they think you may not have done it."

"But you can't tell them I didn't. That's not true."

"No, I won't tell them you did, and I won't tell them you didn't. It's the prosecution's job to prove you did. I just have to create doubt."

"How?"

"Fiction. I want the jury to think your book is a mixture of fact and fiction, and that perhaps the deathbed scene is fiction."

"Roger, you must understand the time has come when everyone should know the truth. Some good must come from all this, and people need to see that we must change the law."

"You can tell the public whatever you like after the trial. Have your day of confession, but not in court. I really don't want you to take the stand."

All evening we debated whether I should testify. He said we can make the final decision after the prosecution completes its evidence.

Over dinner he told me about his godson, Ben, who is only twenty-two and has terminal cancer. Ben has been close to his family since he was born and they are struggling to deal with his imminent death. Roger had informed the court that if Ben died during the trial, he would have to take two days off to attend the funeral and read the eulogy.

After dinner I wanted to go for a long walk to clear my mind before the big day of evidence analysis tomorrow, and Roger insisted on giving me a quick reconnaissance trip so that I wouldn't get lost, especially since it was getting dark.

THE TRIAL

Dunedin High Court: Tuesday 25 October 2011 (Day 1)

I walked to the court with Roger, trying to appear relaxed and confident, as he had trained me to do. Inside, my stomach was churning.

Two prison guards met me at the courthouse door, where my existing bail conditions terminated, and I was escorted down passageways and stairs to an underground area where there were half a dozen prison cells. The inmates were angry, periodically thumping on the doors and making demands of the prison staff.

I had to hand over all of my possessions. I hadn't been warned about this in advance, so my hands and pockets were full: pen and papers, a folder with trial notes, cell phone, car keys, cough mixture and lozenges, and a plastic bag with some crushed biscuits. They took everything, along with my tie and belt, and did a body search.

I pleaded with the correctional office to allow me to keep at least the cough lozenges, because it had become impossible to suppress the irritation in my throat for more than a few minutes. However, the officer in charge was emphatic that I could not keep anything.

"One rule for everyone," he said.

The humiliating journey had begun.

I was alone in the holding cell, a concrete box measuring four meters by three, and I paced, trying to compose myself. Pacing was also the only way to keep warm. There was a concrete bench to sit on, and a neon bulb with a thick plastic protective covering. Below ground level, with no natural light, the cell was cold, damp, and claustrophobic.

Occasionally I stopped pacing and read the abusive graffiti on the walls. Past occupants' expletive-thick protestations of innocence and accusations of police persecution. On one wall POLICE spelt vertically became an acronym for "Police Often Lie In Court Evidence."

I paced and paced. I'm not a murderer. I'm not a criminal. I've done nothing wrong.

An hour went by. I didn't know why there was a delay, but it was very frustrating. I wanted to get on with it.

Eventually Roger was allowed in and explained that there had been a meeting with the judge and the prosecutor, and that I had to come to a follow-up meeting with them. Flanked by two guards, with Roger and the prosecutors some distance behind, I was escorted through the building and upstairs to an old wooden office with an antique table, desk, and paintings. The guards waited at the entrance when I entered the office. Inside, an elegant-looking woman was standing in the middle of the room, and I wondered if she could be the judge.

"Hello, I'm Sean," I said, cautiously. I could hardly say "your honor" in case she was just a court official.

"Good morning. I'm Christine French."

The Last Waltz: Love, Death & Betrayal

I was alone with the judge in her chambers. That didn't seem legally appropriate, but I felt quite at ease, struck by her disarming smile and kindly demeanor. It is rare to perceive a person's compassion and sensitivity so quickly, but this woman definitely had both. I couldn't have hoped for a better judge.

Roger and the two prosecutors joined us and we sat around the table discussing the ground rules for the trial. I made only one contribution.

"Madam Judge, I know it's inappropriate to eat sweets in court, but I have a terrible hacking cough. Would you mind if I discreetly suck cough lozenge's during the trial, please?"

"Of course you may," she replied without hesitation. The prison officers exchanged glances.

At the conclusion of the meeting, the judge said the trial would begin at two pm, after the normal court luncheon break, and I was led back to my cell. This time, all of the cells were full of prisoners waiting for their hearings in the magistrate's court. I must have looked completely out of place in my smart jacket, in contrast to their scruffy clothes. However, a shared adversity bonds people. By lunchtime, the magistrate's court had finished its business for the day and I was alone again.

I continued pacing.

Finally the guards came to lead me up a corridor and through a series of iron doors, locking each one behind us, then ascending a wooden staircase, which led straight into the dock in the middle of the courtroom. Suddenly I was bathed in bright light and surrounded by the imposing architecture of the high court chamber. The contrast was so daunting that I wanted to go back to my dungeon below, but now I was the accused, and at the mercy of the court. I looked around, and it was a relief to see the front row of the public gallery lined with supporters.

The judge entered, the court stood, and the trial began.

Selecting the jury went according to plan. Roger and I thought women would relate better to my situation with Mum, and we got eight out of the twelve – hopefully a good omen. I tried to study them, but I didn't want to get caught doing so, and only glanced their way whenever the judge addressed them directly.

After jury selection, I was asked to plead to the charge of attempted murder. If I don't get to testify, these will be my only spoken words in court.

"Not guilty," I said strongly and confidently. That was easy. I'm not a murderer.

Then there was a procession of medical witnesses, each offering concurring testimony that my mother wanted to die. Some knew about her hunger strike, and they all described how devoted I was to her. There were various accounts of her state of health in the days before she died, and how close she was to death.

During the several breaks in proceedings I was led downstairs to my cell below the court. Even though it was like a dungeon, it became "my" place of solitude and familiarity, and I began looking forward to those steps leading down to it. By contrast, in the courtroom all eyes focused on me. My predicament was made much worse because I couldn't suppress the tickling in my throat, and with each cough all eyes turned to me again. There was nowhere to hide.

I had anticipated a stony-faced, emotionless male judge. Instead, my earlier opinion of Judge French was confirmed during the trial today, and I found myself wondering how such a gentle person could have worked her way up to the top of the cut-throat legal profession. I think of lawyers as specialists at acting out dramas in court, playing games with words and definitions to baffle and deceive juries, while also being more concerned about their own image than justice for their client. Judge French is nothing like that. Several times during the day I caught her eye, and once I thought she gave me a little smile. Time will tell.

I found the day traumatic, although nothing particularly dramatic happened. Before the court adjourned, Roger applied for me to have bail for the night, which the judge granted, with curfew conditions insisted on by the prosecution. I was not allowed to leave my place of residence between seven pm and eight am.

The Last Waltz: Love, Death & Betrayal

Roger and I met briefly at his hotel to analyze the day's events before my curfew.

"It all went very well. It couldn't have gone better," Roger gloated. "All the prosecution witnesses are saying exactly what I want them to. They are playing into my hands."

"I can't see where the prosecution case is," I said.

"It looks pretty thin to me."

We agreed he had won the first day hands down. I should be feeling very relieved, but I'm too overcome with exhaustion. I phoned Raine and told her I may well be home for Christmas.

Later that night

I heard loud banging on the front door. It opened and heavy footsteps followed.

"Stand up! Get out of bed!" the police officer demanded, shining a bright torch in my eyes. "Are you Sean Davison?"

"What on earth are you doing?" I asked.

"Just checking that you're here," he said. "You're on curfew and we'll be checking every night."

"At three am?"

"Get used to it, mate."

It's now five am and I haven't been back to sleep. That intrusion was really unsettling. Why do they have to check in the middle of the night? Why check at all? I came back to the country, after all. I'm hardly going to run away now.

Wednesday 26 October 2011 (Trial, Day 2)

What a bitch!

Mary did it.

That fucking, miserable, manipulative, lying bitch!

There's no doubt about it. In court this morning the police said their Auckland branch received my manuscript anonymously in the post in January 2009. This is the manuscript with Mum's self-portrait on the front cover. Mary's copy. Bitch. This is the same copy the police showed me when they arrested me. I had assumed they had taken it from her – but she sent it to them before my book was published! This explains her email telling me that she was reporting me to the police for murdering Mum.

What the hell was going on in her head?

My sister has put me on trial for murdering Mum. She knew what Mum wanted. She knew I did it for our mother. Bitch. What have I ever done to her? Why? Why would she do this to me? To our family? To Mum's memory? She knew that Mum wanted to die so desperately, and that I was doing Mum's will. Why would she do this to me?

Mum would have never suspected that Mary was capable of such cruelty; otherwise, she would have never have asked me to help her die. No one could have imagined anything so bizarre, that one of my mother's children would try to get another labeled a criminal and incarcerated – for helping carry out her own wishes!

My head's been spinning all morning and I was completely distracted in court. Hope the jury didn't notice. I don't want them to think I'm showing disdain for the court.

I have to put this out of my mind, otherwise I won't make it through the trial... what a conniving, evil, bitch...

Fuck! Fuck! Fuck!

Later the same day

Jindra Tichy was called to the stand after lunch. As she made her way to the witness stand, she turned and gave a knowing glance.

The prosecutor began with the standard question.

"Dr. Tichy, please tell the court how you know the accused."

"I want to say from the start that I don't like Sean's mother. She's a terrible woman for asking Sean to help her to die. It wasn't right."

I quickly scribbled a note to Roger: "Ask her if she ever met my mother. She didn't!"

"Will you answer the question, Dr. Tichy?" insisted the prosecutor.

"And Sean is a fool, and I've told him that before."

The Last Waltz: Love, Death & Betrayal

She then took the court by the scruff of its neck and continued to ask and answer her own questions to highlight what she believed the court should know. She said that I was her very best friend and that I had taken great care of her own mother for four months when I visited her in Czechoslovakia – and she had survived. I could see the judge was intrigued by Jindra's performance and seemed visibly moved by her account of me looking after her mother.

Jindra was great. She wasn't going to dance to the tune of a prosecutor wanting to send her best friend to jail. During her testimony, I noticed the prosecutor and Roger, through an exchange of glances, mutually agreeing not to proceed with this witness. They stood and said they had no further questions. Jindra puffed out her chest and strode confidently from the witness box, turning my way and giving a little wink as she passed.

Ian was called. It was surreal to see my best friend in the box as a compliant prosecution witness, albeit a carefully trained one. He stuck to the agreed script. He recounted how he had followed my mother's decline closely and gave a most complete description of her state of health and mind. He also described his insight into my terrible dilemma. He made it very clear that my mother was desperate, knew what she wanted, and wanted me to help her. He came across as sensitive and intelligent.

Roger then cross-examined him.

"Mr. Landreth, what are your views on assisted suicide?"

"Do you mean what are my views on youth in Asia?"

"No, what are your views on assisted suicide?"

"Sorry, you've got me there."

Later the same day

"Day two to us, Sean," Roger proclaimed again, when we met at his hotel. "It's going very well, couldn't have been better."

"I couldn't take in much," I said. "I lost focus after Mary's bombshell."

"I had everything under control. Got the prosecution tripping all over themselves."

We briefly discussed what Fergus might say tomorrow. He will be interviewed via a satellite feed first thing in the morning. Roger's not sure what angle the prosecution will take with him, though we're both concerned about the way his statement was tampered with. Still, Fergus will only tell the truth, so I can't see that it matters what's in his statement.

Later the same day

"Thanks, Ian, your testimony was really good, very convincing. You had the jury wiping their eyes when you described my mother asking you to make sure I helped her."

"I was disappointed not to get my youth-in-Asia joke in, but I have some fantastic news for you."

"I like good news."

"I recognized a woman on the jury – I thought I was bound to know someone on it. It gets better. This person has often spoken to me about your situation, long before she was selected for the jury, and there's no way she will ever find you guilty!"

"That really is fantastic news. We've definitely got it in the bag, then."

"Shall I casually pop by her place tonight – with chocolates?"

Ian's jauntiness is a tonic.

Later that night (2 am)

"Are you Sean Davison?" demanded the police officer while shining the torch in my face.

"Yes, I still am."

"Just checking."

I couldn't sleep before the police came because I was anxiously waiting for them, and now I can't sleep because they've visited. It's a good thing I'm not taking the stand today, as I'd be a total zombie.

The Last Waltz: Love, Death & Betrayal

The police surprise about Mary sending them the manuscript doesn't help. Perhaps it's really that that's stopping me from sleeping. God – what a bitch... Why? Why?

Thursday 27 October 2011 (Trial, Day 3)

I wasn't with it again today, just too tired, but it didn't matter.

Unfortunately Roger wasn't with it, either, and that did matter. His godson died today. He heard at lunchtime, and after that his mind was definitely not on my case. The police presented masses of evidence and heaps of witnesses, but he barely raised his voice. I'm sorry for his loss, but this is a disaster for me. I hope the jury don't think we're throwing in the towel.

Before he received the news about his godson, the court heard Fergus's testimony, live from London. Fergus kept squirming in his chair and gave the impression he really didn't want to be there. He probably didn't.

I thought the balance of his evidence helped me, because he explained that when he left New Zealand two days before Mum died, her health was stable and her mind sound. He agreed with Roger that Mum was perfectly capable of saying she didn't want to have the morphine cocktail I gave her, or of simply turning her head away if offered the glass. This all helped highlight the obvious fact that Mum made the decision to end her life, not me. Fortunately, the issue of the police changing Fergus's written statement was no longer relevant, since he was giving evidence in person. Good grief, that would have opened up a whole new can of worms.

The judge adjourned the trial until Tuesday, so that Roger can go home for the funeral, which is actually a welcome respite for me. It's so very intense in the court, in the dock. And today wasn't a good day, as the police released all their evidence from my laptop. Obviously, I knew what was there, but it was very embarrassing having my personal diaries read out in court, and some passages must have been chosen to cause as much humiliation as possible. Mary must be loving this.

The Last Waltz: Love, Death & Betrayal

My diary said many times that I didn't think any jury in New Zealand could find me guilty of any crime for helping my mother to her death. The judge looked at me. I'm sure she winked.

Supporter numbers are growing every day, and they hang around after the trial so they can offer encouragement and advise as I leave.

Later the same day

"Definitely our day again, Sean," Roger concluded back at his hotel. "All that stuff on your laptop was supporting you. Don't know why they read out some of it."

"Some of the jury were in tears, which must be a good sign," I said.

"Indeed they were. You may have noticed I kept looking straight at them and pausing at particularly moving moments, when I cross-examined the witness. I wanted to let them soak it up," he boasted.

"And I liked the way you were being so friendly with the prison guards. The jury notice this kind of thing, and they can see you aren't the average criminal."

Roger is putting a brave face on it, but he really is grieving over the death of his godson. He'll be on a plane back to Hamilton tonight. We still haven't made a decision about whether I should testify or not. I suppose it's my decision. I shouldn't keep deflecting it onto Roger.

At least the judge lifted my night-time curfew. She was clearly not impressed when Roger informed her about my early-morning harassment from the police. I'll sleep better tonight, perhaps.

Friday 28 October 2011

I'm having a complete break today.

Apart from discovering that Mary's an absolute and incomprehensible bitch, life's good and the trial really couldn't be going better.

Hell, won't Mary be disappointed if I walk free next week. Not just free, but victorious.

The Last Waltz: Love, Death & Betrayal

This trial has highlighted the absurdity of my arrest and prosecution, and I'm finally feeling it was all worth it. Of course I shouldn't count my chickens just yet, but even Roger is confident we have it in the bag.

I wonder what Mary's thinking now...

Does she really want me to go to jail? Or does she regret it and think she went too far? No, she's gloating. She's loving every moment.

Sunday 30 October 2011

Most of the leading papers in the country have run editorials supporting me and the need to change the law. Editorials supposedly reflect the views of their readers, so this is a good sign. The only exception was the *Otago Daily Times* editorial, so I hope it doesn't reflect the views of the jury. Actually, some of the reporting in the *Otago Daily Times* this week was shocking and sensational. Evidently a trainee reporter was standing in while the regular court reporter was on vacation. What bad timing!

Monday 31 October 2011

I took a long walk on the Otago Peninsula. I'm feeling very relaxed and confident. I've put a lot of thought into whether to take the stand or not, and I've decided I won't.

It seems so strange coming to this point, when I've been waiting more than a year for my day in court, to explain my actions and convince the jury that I did not commit a crime. Over the past year, I've had so many reflective walks up Table Mountain in the evening twilight, contemplating what I would say, how I would say it, and the peace it would bring me. But now that the moment has come, I realize it would not be wise to take the stand. Roger says the prosecutor would keep me there for several days, dissecting the incriminating words in my manuscript line by line. But the deciding factor is that if I take the stand, I will have to expose the lies told by other people to protect me. Not just the ones who gave court testimony, but those who gave written statements, as well.

The Last Waltz: Love, Death & Betrayal

Over the first three days of the trial, the evidence from the district nurses who visited Mum were so contradictory that it was obvious some were trying to cover for me. One nurse said my mother was so near death that she couldn't even swallow water, implying that she probably died of natural causes. Another nurse who visited the same day said Mum was alert and could easily drink water if the glass was held for her.

And all of the other people who signed statements saying that I hadn't told them how I helped my mother die, could be exposed as committing perjury. And Jindra will look a fool if I have to tell the court that she did open my email attachment and we did discuss my mother's death. And, of course, there's Jo. I can't expose my sister's loyalty either.

So many good people have tried to protect me. Now I must protect them with my silence. I am having my day in court, but I won't have my day on the stand.

Tuesday 1 November 2011 (Trial, Day 4)

Oh, fuck! Total disaster. I'm in an impossible situation. The trial resumed behind closed doors today, and the prosecution just socked it to us.

The day began well, with Roger filing to have the case thrown out. It's called a section 347. He told the court that I had no charge to answer. However, after behind-the-scenes discussions with the prosecutor, he withdrew this application and accepted that the trial had to continue.

Then things got really good. The judge herself filed a section 347 and said she believed I had no charge to answer. I couldn't believe my luck. The nightmare was as good as over... if only the day could have stopped there.

But wham! The prosecution roared in with guns blazing, probably believing they had no choice but to show their hand in case the judge ended the trial. The two prosecutors really turned up the heat by focusing on my manuscript, analyzing line by line the days before Mum died. They chose single phrases to indicate that my mother's death at the very end was not in her hands, but in mine. They argued

The Last Waltz: Love, Death & Betrayal

that although she had made it clear in previous weeks that she wanted to die, the actual moment of her death was chosen unilaterally by me, and this clearly fitted the legal description of attempted murder.

After several hours of discussion about legal precedents, the judge said she had no choice but to keep the attempted murder charge before the jury. However, the prosecution agreed to add an alternative charge of assisted suicide.

Roger had previously explained why this wasn't the original charge, but now it seems the prosecution gets two bites of the cake. If they don't succeed with one, then they will succeed with the other.

As usual, we went to his hotel to analyze what had happened. Roger collapsed in an armchair, tie undone, shirt untucked – he looked a mess.

"If this goes to the jury, you will be found guilty of attempted murder. There's no doubt. None," he said. "You have to plead guilty to assisted suicide."

"But Roger, surely the prosecution can't convince ten of the twelve that I tried to murder Mum. I've seen the sympathy on their faces. Some even cried."

"Sympathy's not what counts. They'll be directed by the judge to follow the legal definition of attempted murder."

"But I didn't murder ..."

"Sean, today, from your own manuscript, diary, and letters, came an avalanche of confessions of what the law defines as 'attempted murder.' Plead guilty to assisted suicide tomorrow, then the jury will be discharged and it goes straight to sentencing."

"If the prosecution are positive they've got me for attempted murder, why the alternative charge?"

"Hedging their bets. If the jury were to acquit you on attempted murder, they would definitely accept assisted suicide."

"So the prosecution has doubt."

"You can't be certain with juries."

"Then we should go to the jury."

"Sean, I am your lawyer and I am advising you to plead guilty to assisted suicide because I believe if this goes to the jury you will be convicted of attempted murder. Unless you're determined to go down in a blaze of glory for the sake of your euthanasia supporters, you must plead guilty."

"What? I'm not doing this for my supporters! This is happening to *me*!" My heart was pounding so loudly I could barely get the words out.

"Then think of your family. Do they want you in jail?"

"I need time to think."

"Look, Sean, go climb a mountain or whatever it is you do, and come back and tell me you're pleading guilty."

"Can't I tell you in the morning?"

"The judge needs to know tonight so she can prepare her direction to the jury if you're not pleading guilty."

"I have to decide now so as not to inconvenience the judge?"

"You don't want to annoy her," he said. "The other thing you need to be aware of is that the assisted suicide charge is for 'inciting, procuring and counseling' a suicide. It's the only charge that fits your case."

Later the same day

In the eyes of the law, in 21st century New Zealand, I am guilty of murdering Mum. Most people are unaware of assisted suicide unless they face it in their own lives. The only thing I knew was that I must free Mum from her agony – and that that was the right thing to do.

I certainly don't regret that. I think any humane person would have done what I did, in the same circumstances.

And now if I don't accept the inciting charge, I will be convicted of attempted murder and go to jail, which means my boys will grow up with a father who has served time for murder. And the public will wonder what really went on in Mum's room that night and suspect me of something.

I have to make a decision by the morning. Roger wants it tonight, but bugger that, he can wait. How could I have thought it was simple?

The Last Waltz: Love, Death & Betrayal

Ross Creek: later

It's after midnight. I have walked and walked and talked and talked. I'm trying to talk myself out of tomorrow.

I had a sleep by the reservoir and dreamt I heard your voice, Mum, saying to me there is no choice.

That's not enough. I can take the truth. Tell me what I must do. I'll stay awake till I hear you.

That night you died, our night, there was no choice, but I don't understand what you mean when you say that there's no choice now.

Do I plead guilty of inciting your suicide? That's as bad as murder. I can't live with that.

You came to me before. I am listening now. Tell me what to do.

Later

I was at home with Mum for many years. She had given up work until all her children were at school, and I was the youngest. Those earliest memories are the ones I treasure most. By necessity, she took me everywhere. She was so loving. She always made me feel that each trip was all about me. She never hit me, and I was rarely scolded. A mother's love is so pure and unconditional.

Later

The stars are fading. The sun will rise soon. But I think it's setting on me.

Mum has given me no answers, though I begged for help.

What happens today will define my life forever. Do I leave my destiny in the hands of the jury?

Wednesday 2 November 2011 (Trial, Day 5)

The dungeon was cold, damp, and dark. I'd never felt so alone. Mum deserted me in my hour of greatest need. I sat and stared at the walls, lost in defeat. I know that I've done no wrong.

The Last Waltz: Love, Death & Betrayal

I was led up to the gallows by the prison guards, who were quiet and sullen. There was a sense of impending doom.

I sat in the dock while the court waited for the judge. The jury sat and stared, searching my face for answers. They knew nothing about yesterday's closed-door meeting, but sensed something was going to happen.

The judge entered. The court rose. She looked tired. Had she read my book? Did she understand my story. What if she has to ask her son what my mother asked me? Would she want him to end up here?

Judge French read the alternative charge.

"Mr. Davison, you are charged with inciting, procuring, and counseling the assisted suicide of Patricia Elizabeth Davison on 25 October 2006. How do you plead?"

What a terrible dilemma. No son should have to go through this.

"Mum do you really want to die tonight?" I tried to collect myself. I thought and thought. I knew the answer to the question I was posing myself. I said, "I promise you, Mum, your wish to die will come true tonight."

Her eyes lit up. "What?" It was as if she finally heard what I had been saying.

"Mum, you deserve to die. You don't deserve this suffering."

She quickly agreed. "Yes." She clearly believed there had been some injustice in the way her life had been prolonged. She then affirmed, "I want to die tonight. I feel dreadful. I feel pain everywhere, and I can hardly talk."

There was no doubt now. I prepared what I calculated would be a lethal drink of crushed morphine tablets. I held it in front of her and said, "If you drink this, you will die." I wanted to be sure, absolutely sure, that there was no hesitation.

She answered, "You are a wonderful son."

I said, "It is not how you planned it. It is not what I planned. This is an event that will live long after you die. Do you want me to help you die?"

The Last Waltz: Love, Death & Betrayal

"No one will ever know." No one need ever know, that was true, but I would. Her destiny was not in her hands, as she'd planned, but in mine.

I held the glass to her lips and gently poured the liquid into her mouth.

"You are a wonderful son."

I have no choice. I must do what's right. I choked for air. "Guilty," I mumbled, the word barely audible.

"Guilty?" the judge asked. I could only nod.

"This is an event that will live long after you die."

"No one will ever know."

We all come to crucial markers in our lives, points that define our lives forever. From that moment on, everything in one's life is counted either before or after that marker. I had come to that place. For the rest of my days, my life will be defined by what happened before and after the night Mum died.

"The court convicts you of counseling and procuring the suicide of Patricia Elizabeth Davison. You are remanded on bail to appear in court on November 24 for sentencing," the judge announced. "Court dismissed."

Roger took me aside before we left the court. "Remember what I told you, Sean. I want you pumping your fists in the air as we leave the court," he said. "This is what the media wants to see, it's what the public wants to see."

"But we lost."

"No, this was a great victory, Sean. I got you off of the attempted murder charge." he said. "Victory, victory. Come and tell the media how happy you feel."

Sure enough, the reporters were outside the door. They quickly fired questions: How do you feel? Are you pleased to get out of the attempted murder charge? What about your job? What has this done for the cause?

"Thank you for your questions and concern." I said. "Some people will say that today's verdict is a victory, but for me, my family, and the memory of my mother, it is a terrible tragedy." Roger slunk into the background.

And they don't even know of the second tragedy – that Mary's actions have forever torn our family apart.

The Last Waltz: Love, Death & Betrayal

Later the same day

I visited Roger in his hotel room tonight because he's leaving early in the morning. He wasn't his normal self. Perhaps he was drained from the trial, and perhaps he was relieved that it was over. I'm sure he's still suffering from the death of his godson.

We chatted for an hour or so. His veneer had gone and he told me about his own upbringing and complex family dynamics. It was the first time I'd seen him truly in touch with his feelings. We didn't discuss the trial at all. What was done was done, and there was no need to scratch the wound tonight.

THREE WEEKS LATER

Wednesday 23 November 2011

Dear Sean,

I have sent off a character statement to urge the judge to show clemency.
We pray that things go well with you at the sentencing and you will be back soon.
You have conducted yourself with dignity.
God be with you.
Much love and blessings.
Arch

Dear Archbishop,

Thank you for your kindness in writing to the judge.
I wish I could find the answers in your Christian God, but alas I can't.
Sean

Dear Sean

I have never said that God is a Christian.
Answers can be found in many places.
God be with you.
Love, Arch

Is this my freedom? Is this the difference between jail and justice? I have to stay focused. This is only an email, and Archbishop Tutu is just a man.

No! He's not just a man! He's Archbishop Desmond Tutu – a Nobel peace laureate and one of the most respected spokespersons for our humanity. When he speaks, the world listens. Surely, no judge in the world would send me to jail after a request for leniency by the "The Arch."

Would they?

Or is this my last day of freedom? Tomorrow I could be in jail, or under house arrest. The uncertainty is driving me crazy.

Well-wishers have been phoning all morning, full of good cheer, and almost everyone is confident that I won't go to jail. If I get a house arrest sentence, most think it will be a three-month slap on the wrist. Roger says to be prepared for a more standard six months.

Me? I think I might well walk free. Judge French is compassionate and has done what the law requires by convicting me, but I think she will use her judicial discretion in sentencing. She must be aware that the vast majority of people want to see the law on voluntary euthanasia changed and have no desire to see me punished. So I'm quietly confident I will be a free man tomorrow night – though one with a criminal record.

Perhaps I shouldn't have been so optimistic when I spoke to Raine yesterday, in case things go badly. At the moment, she's preparing for my imminent return to resume nappy-changing and bedtime storytelling duties.

I will try to sleep now. I could have a cellmate tomorrow night.

SENTENCING

Dunedin High Court: Thursday 24 November 2011

It's a glorious morning with bright sunlight sparkling from wet surfaces after last night's rain. I had breakfast with the first glimmer of dawn, then packed my bags, wondering the whole time where I will be tonight. The unknown is the

The Last Waltz: Love, Death & Betrayal

hardest thing to deal with, and I can't ignore the fact that prison is on the cards. Here on the patio, with my laptop and a strong coffee, I'm soaking up every sight, sound, and smell, conscious that this could be my last taste, for a while, of life as a free man.

I savored each breath of free air as I walked down Moray Place, passing a handful of journalists and a TV camera outside the court. There were a few supporters gathering at the entrance, some wearing *"Every mum should have a Sean"* T-shirt.

Inside the courthouse door, two prison officers escorted me to the underground dungeon and then conducted the standard frisk, before leading me into my cell.

There was a clunk from the heavy iron door, and the key was turned.

Alone again, I removed my shoes and took Mum's photo from inside one sock and the adhesive putty from the other sock. I had a thick black crayon tucked under my toes, with which I defiantly wrote on the wall: "No mum should need a Sean."

Above this I stuck the photo. It was an old black and white picture of five-year-old me sitting on Mum's knee. I looked happy and innocent; she looked refined and beautiful. That was how we started, and though today I am to be judged, we'd already passed the test that matters. I was there for her as she knew I would be, and both of us knew that what we did was right on that fateful night. On the most fundamental level, we maintained our honor and integrity, and on that level we had nothing to fear.

But the wheels of justice grind on. I was escorted from the holding cell to the courtroom to listen to, first, the prosecutor insisting I should go to jail for committing a premeditated crime, and then my defender's plea for leniency, which culminated in his reading Archbishop Tutu's letter and consequent gasps of excitement. Even God made his presence felt, it seemed. Dramatic theater at its very best.

The court fell silent, waiting for the judge to pronounce sentencing.

The Last Waltz: Love, Death & Betrayal

The judge spoke: The law is the law; I had not appreciated it; my crime was premeditated, and I had shown no remorse.

"I start my calculation of sentence at twenty-four months' imprisonment." There were gasps from the gallery.

"I reduce it by twenty per cent for pleading guilty at the first opportunity." *(That leaves about twenty-one months. Shit!)*

"I reduce it by twenty per cent for no previous convictions." *(God, that's still about eighteen months!)*

And something else for something else... my mind was everywhere.

"Now that your sentence is reduced to twelve months' imprisonment, you qualify for home detention. I sentence you to five months' home detention."

Five months? Five months? Is that good or bad? I can't get my mind around it. It's just a number, a number that I hadn't considered. Six months was the absolute worst, three months a likely figure – but five, what does five mean?

No prison. That's good. How do I reconcile myself to this five-month sentence?

The court adjourned. I was in the box, surrounded by court officials with bits of paper to sign, while supporters hovered in the background. They seemed to be in shock, so perhaps I should be, too.

The court gave instructions for me to be taken directly to my house of arrest, where I would be met by probation services to have an ankle bracelet fitted. On the way out, I looked around to soak up my final moments of freedom. This was the last time I would see a crowded street for five months, the last time I would see so many people for five months, the last time I would breathe free air for five months.

Later - At John's house

I am by myself. The sun is shining. I've walked around and studied every room – several times. This view is my life for the next five months, but I am at peace. I did the right thing.

The Last Waltz: Love, Death & Betrayal

This part of my life, this part right here, this is called destiny.

The Last Waltz: Love, Death & Betrayal

The Most Reverend Desmond M Tutu, O.M.S.G. D.D. F.K.C.
Anglican Archbishop Emeritus of Cape Town

PO Box 1092, Milnerton, Cape Town 7435
Suite 43, Frazzitta Business Park, cnr Freedom Way & Koeberg Road, Milnerton 7441
Tel: (+27) 021 552 7524
Fax: (+27) 021 552 7529
E-mail: mpilo@iafrica.com

24 November 2011

To: The New Zealand High Court

Character Reference: Dr. Sean Davison

Although I respect the law in New Zealand I feel that the case of Dr. Sean Davison is an exceptional and tragic one. In my opinion he is an upright citizen who has made a contribution to society and has much more to offer. In South Africa he worked in a laboratory which was instrumental in identifying the remains of anti-apartheid activists whose mass grave sites were revealed during the TRC hearings which I chaired.

I urge the court to show leniency in sentencing Sean Davison.

Desmond

Archbishop Emeritus Desmond Tutu
Cape Town, South Africa

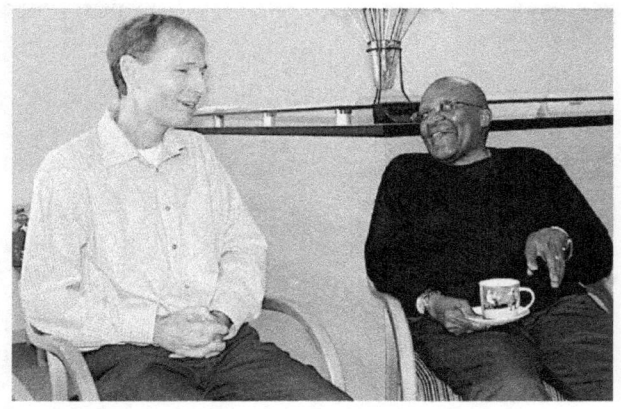

Sean thanks Archbishop Desmond Tutu for his support (June 2012).

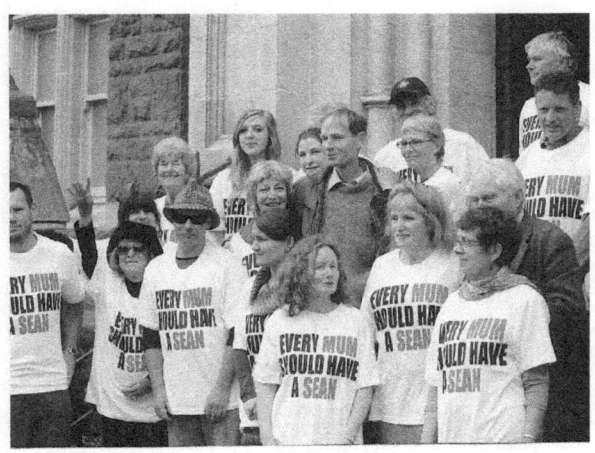

Sean with supporters outside the High Court in Dunedin.

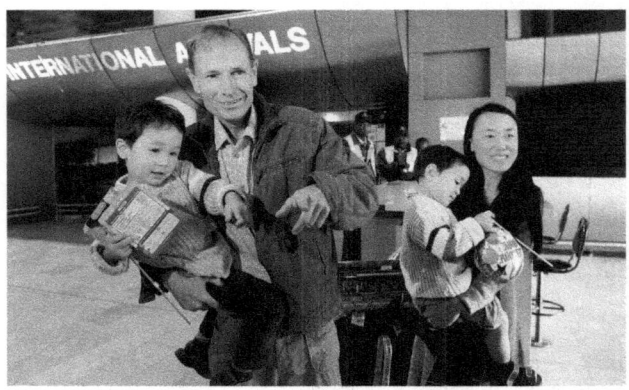

May 2012: Raine, Flynn and Finn welcome Sean at Cape Town International Airport.

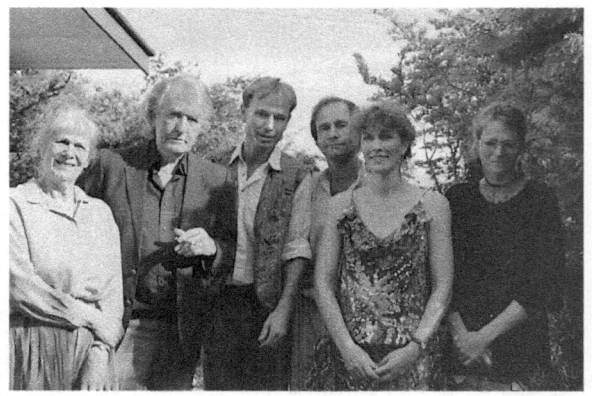

Family Reunion 1994: Pat, Paddy, Sean, Fergus, Mary and Jo.

www.ingramcontent.com/pod-product-compliance
Lightning Source LLC
Chambersburg PA
CBHW032249150426
43195CB00008BA/381